Rheumatology of the Lower Limbs in Clinical Practice

José António Pereira da Silva
Anthony D. Woolf

Rheumatology of the Lower Limbs in Clinical Practice

Springer

Dr. José António Pereira da Silva
MD, PhD
Department of Rheumatology
University Hospital
Coimbra
Portugal

Dr. Anthony D. Woolf, MSc, MBBS
FRCP
Department of Rheumatology
Royal Cornwall Hospital
Truro
United Kingdom

First published in 2010 as part of Rheumatology in Practice
(ISBN 978-1-84882-580-2)

Rheumatology in Practice (ISBN 978-1-84882-580-2) was previously published in Portuguese by **Diagnósteo** as *Reumatologia Prática* by José António Pereira da Silva, 2005.

ISBN 978-1-4471-2252-4 e-ISBN 978-1-4471-2253-1
DOI 10.1007/978-1-4471-2253-1
Springer London Dordrecht Heidelberg New York

British Library Cataloguing in Publication Data
A catalogue record for this book is available from the British Library

Library of Congress Control Number: 2011944228

Printed on acid-free paper

Springer is part of Springer Science+Business Media (www.springer.com)

Contents

GUIDE

TYPICAL CASES

MAIN POINTS

UNDERLINED

TABLES

Chapter 1
Regional Syndromes

Low Back Pain

Low back pain is the most common complaint after the common cold. Almost everyone has at least one episode of low back pain during their lives. In the USA, it accounts for around 3% of all visits to doctors.

Low back pain often takes the form of an acute episode which occurs most commonly between the ages of 30 and 50. About 90% of episodes of acute backache clear up in less than 8 weeks regardless of the treatment. A small minority of people will, however, have recurring acute attacks or their condition will become chronic, with considerable pain and disability. Chronic low back pain is an important public health problem with a significant social and economic impact involving substantial direct and indirect costs.

In most cases of chronic mechanical back pain, it is impossible to make a precise diagnosis because of the complexity of the structures in question and the multiplicity of potential factors. The course of chronic back pain is closely related to psychological and social factors that are difficult to assess. Even in these cases, however, we can arrive at an approximate diagnosis that enables us to help the patient.

Only a small percentage of cases involve a specific etiology requiring special diagnostic and therapeutic action, but it is precisely these cases that require our attention most. Low back pain may be the first manifestation of a potentially fatal disease.

J.A.P. da Silva, A.D. Woolf, *Rheumatology of the Lower Limbs in Clinical Practice*, DOI 10.1007/978-1-4471-2253-1_1,

The approach to patients with low back pain has three main goals:

1. Preventing acute episodes from becoming chronic
2. Identifying cases requiring specific treatment (red flags)
3. Relieving the symptoms and, in particular, improving the patient's physical and social functions while avoiding unnecessary tests

Functional Anatomy

The functional anatomy of the lumbar spine is very similar to that already described for the cervical spine: a set of five vertebrae one on top of the other separated by intervertebral discs.

Posteriorly, pedicles project on either side of the vertebral body. The transverse processes extend laterally from them. The upper and lower joint surfaces that extend from the pedicles, form facet joints with the adjacent vertebrae. The alignment of the lumbar facet joints is almost anteroposterior, which is why they are capable only of flexion and extension. Rotation of the torso depends, therefore, on the thoracic spine.

The lumbar spinal canal contains and protects the end of the spinal cord (the medullary cone ends at approximately L1/L2) and the nerve roots forming the cauda equina. The first lumbar root emerges between L1 and L2 and so on (Fig. 1.1).

The vertebrae and their joints are stabilized by a large number of ligaments, which may be the site of back pain-causing lesions, but are impossible to evaluate separately either clinically or by imaging. These ligaments and their insertions are common targets of pathology in ankylosing spondylitis and the other seronegative spondyloarthropathies.

The lumbar spine is mobilized by muscles running along the vertebral grooves, which have multiple insertions along the posterior aspect of the spine. The nerve roots and regional nerve branches are located between these muscles. They may all be the site of disease but cannot be examined individually.

Some aspects require closer attention.

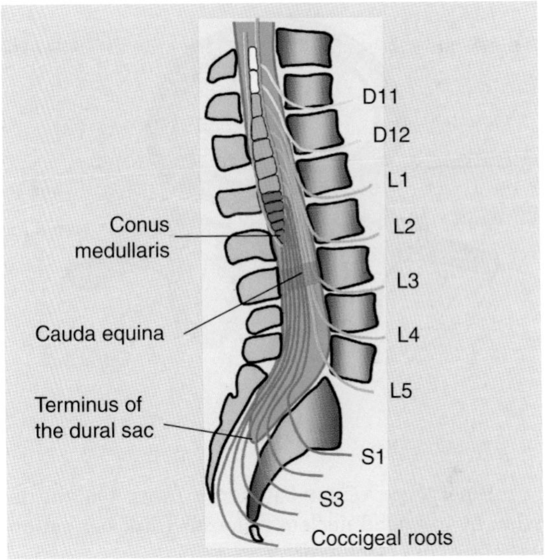

FIGURE 1.1 Emergence of lumbar, sacral and coccigeal nerve roots

The intervertebral foramen through which the nerve roots emerge is limited anteriorly by the intervertebral disk, which may herniate, compressing the root and leading to neurogenic pain (e.g. sciatica) (Fig. 1.2). Posteriorly, the nerve roots are in contact with the facet joint. This is a synovial joint that is frequently affected by osteoarthritis, often with exuberant osteophytes. These osteophytes may cause compression of the root just like a herniated disk, and usually the symptoms are indistinguishable.

The lumbar spinal canal houses the roots that innervate the lower limbs and sacral region. In some people it can be constitutionally narrow. The canal may be reduced further by spondylolisthesis (when a vertebral body slides over the one below it), by prolapsed disks or by large osteophytes from the intervertebral joints. Neural tumors, such as neurofibroma or meningioma are Disk herniation less common causes. When the canal is markedly narrowed, the roots may be compressed to the point of dysfunction, causing pain and weakness in the

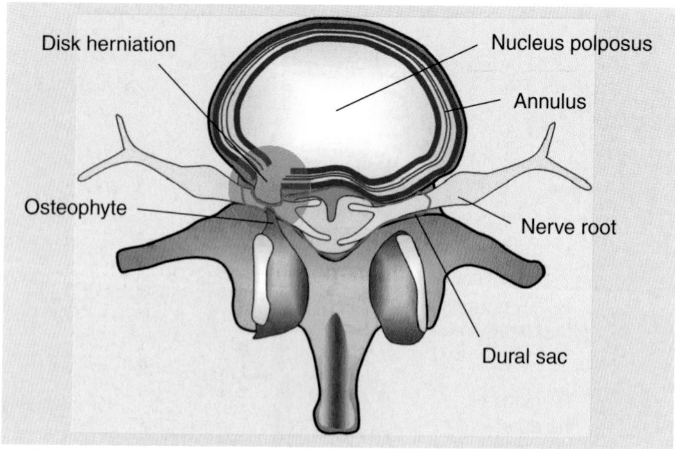

FIGURE 1.2 Emergence of lumbar nerve roots. On the left side: compression by extruded nucleus polposus (disk herniation) or by osteophytes from the facet joint

Osteophyte area served by that root or diffuse exercise-dependent pain (claudication) and neurological deficit affecting the lower limbs (lumbar stenosis) or only the sacral roots (cauda equina syndrome).

Radiological Anatomy

In an anteroposterior x-ray (Fig. 1.3) the alignment of the vertebrae may be seen. Malalignment is called scoliosis. Look for lytic lesions (the "disappearance" of a pedicle or a tranverse process may be the only sign of a metastasis). Note the regularity of the intervertebral spaces and the articular borders as well as the presence of osteophytes or syndesmophytes. The facet joints of the lower vertebrae can, at times, be seen in this projection.

On the lateral film (Fig. 1.4) we get a better idea of the morphology of the vertebral bodies (crush fractures, osteophytes, or squaring of the anterior border) and the size of the

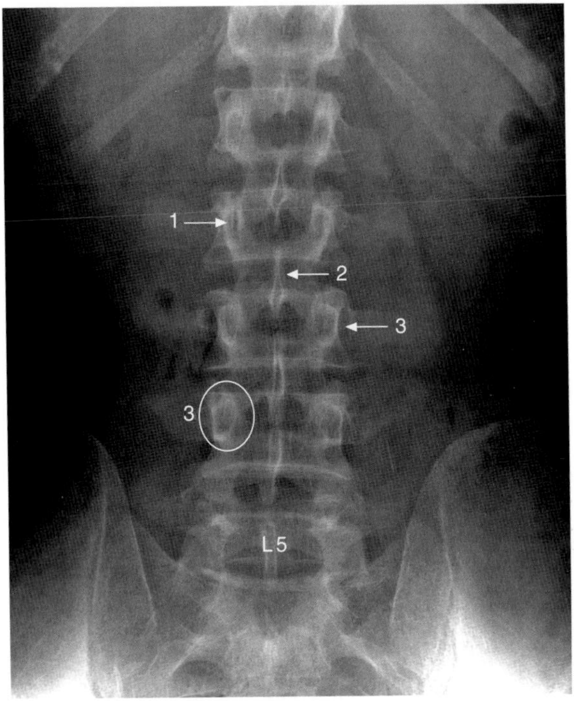

FIGURE 1.3 Lumbar spine radiograph: antero-posterior view. *1* Facet joint. *2* Projection of the spinous process. *3* Projection of the pedicle

intervertebral spaces (i.e. the disc spaces): they increase slightly from L1 to L4 (L4–L5 is generally covered by the iliac bone). Look at the regularity and density of the vertebral platforms. Look for any accentuation or reduction of the normal lordosis.

Look for any calcification of the intervertebral disks or ligaments. Assess the contrast in density between the vertebral body and the neighboring tissue, as a reduction may indicate osteoporosis. Do not mistake the superimposition of intestinal gas for a lytic lesion. Spondylolisthesis is clearly seen in this projection (anterior dislocation of a vertebra over the one below).

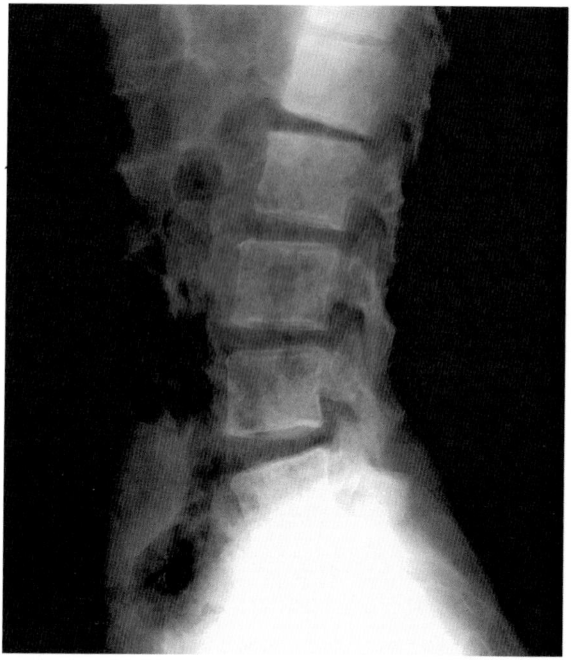

FIGURE 1.4 Lumbar spine radiograph: lateral view

Common Causes of Low Back Pain

The most common causes of low back pain are shown in Table 1.1. Almost all cases will fall into one of the first three categories. Our main goal is to distinguish them from the others and treat them all as effectively as possible.

The Enquiry

How and when did it start?

Pain that appears for the first time before the age of 30 or after 50 requires attention, as it is much more likely to

TABLE 1.1 Common causes of low back pain and suggestive manifestations and alarm signals

Nature of the problem	Suggestive manifestations
Acute mechanical low back pain	Acute pain Paravertebral muscle spasm Young patient
Chronic mechanical low back pain	Chronic, recurring mechanical pain No systemic manifestations No neurological signs
Fibromyalgia	Generalized pain No limitations to mobility Diffuse tenderness on palpation of the paravertebral (and other) muscles
Spondylodiscitis	ALARM SIGNALS ("red flags")!
Sacroiliitis	Inflammatory low back pain
Metastases	Localized pain
Referred pain	Nocturnal pain
Interspinous ligamentitis	Fever, weight loss,...
Neurological compromise	History of neoplasm
Osteoporotic fracture	Associated visceral manifestations Risk or evidence of osteoporosis Onset before age 30 or after 50 Neurological manifestations Limitation of movement in all directions

be due to a specific condition. The same goes for an acute change in the characteristics of chronic back pain.

The onset of muscle spasm, sciatica and osteoporotic fractures is usually sudden and related to flexion or forced rotation. The onset of inflammatory, infectious or even metastatic lesions is progressive, reaching its peak in a few weeks or months.

Conversely, patients with common, chronic back pain usually go to the doctor after months or years of suffering with recurrent, intense episodes superimposed.

Where is the pain? Does it radiate?

The location of the pain can tell us a lot.

The more precise the location of the pain, the more likely a specific diagnosis.

Chronic backache and the pain caused by fibromyalgia tend to be diffuse and imprecisely located. On the other hand, in discitis, metastasis or osteoporotic fracture,the patient usually identifies a focal painful area. Pain due to sacroiliitis is felt mainly in the sacrolumbar region, radiating to the buttocks.

The location of the pain can also suggest the origin of referred pain (Fig. 1.5).

The patient should always be asked about radiation of the pain, paresthesia and its distribution, disturbances of the sphincters or localized weakness.

Pain radiating along a dermatome suggests radicular compression. The most common of these conditions is so-called *sciatica*, which is caused by irritation of the L5 and/or S1 roots. Paresthetic pain radiates down the outer aspect of the thigh, down the leg and may reach the foot. Compression of roots higher up is rare.

A description of weakness in the legs is very common in back-pain patients and should not be ignored if the neurological examination confirms it.

What is the rhythm of the pain?

In most cases the pain will be typically mechanical, i.e. it is worse with movement (flexion and extension, walking or standing upright) and is alleviated at rest, especially lying down. Obesity and increased lumbar lordosis are often present.

Any inflammatory pain requires special attention. It is an alarm signal. Low back pain that persists or predominates at night, with or without morning stiffness, means,

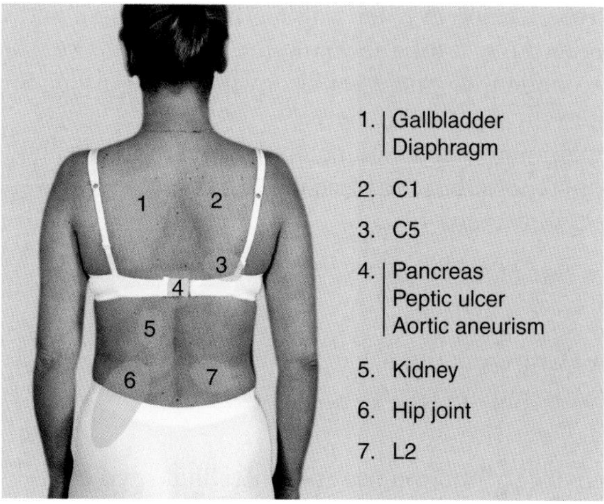

FIGURE 1.5 Areas of pain referred to the lumbar and gluteal areas

until proven otherwise, an inflammatory condition (spondylitis, spondylodiscitis,...), metastasis (breast, prostate, kidney,...) or osteoporotic fracture.

What exacerbates or relieves the pain?

We have already mentioned exercise, but there are other aspects that also deserve our attention. Pain that is alleviated by movement is probably related to an inflammatory process. Exacerbation of the pain by Valsava's maneuvers (deliberate or when coughing, sneezing or defecating, for example) suggests nerve root irritation, especially if there is typical radiation. Patients with radiculopathy often also say that the pain is more intense when they are standing still than when they are walking.

Lumbar stenosis, which is more common in the elderly, is associated with a suggestive, but not always clear, clinical pattern. The pain is deep, diffuse and ill defined (like "tiredness"), involving the lumbar region and the proximal part of the limbs. It worsens when walking and may be dysesthetic.

As a rule, it appears after walking for some time and forces the patient to rest for a few minutes. The pain is usually more intense when the patient walks downhill than uphill. Strange, isn't it? Why should that be?[1]

Impairment of the sphincters is rare and appears late in lumbar stenosis, but the patient often complains of weakness in the lower limbs.

The systematic enquiry

> An alarm signal in a back-pain patient makes the systematic enquiry particularly important.

Signs of peptic, pancreatic, intestinal, gynecological or urological disease can be the key to diagnosis. A description of psoriasis may reinforce the possibility of psoriatic spondylitis, etc.

We must ask about important constitutional symptoms like fever or weight loss if we have not already done so.

Psychological and Social Evaluation

These aspects are particularly important in a context of chronic, mechanical low back pain. Indeed, it has been shown that the patient's psychological profile is one of the most decisive factors in determining whether an acute episode evolves into a chronic condition. The patient's convictions as to the nature and prognosis of the disease and the ways of dealing with the problem (coping strategies) are decisive elements that we must consider. Labor or legal disputes (e.g. suing for compensation after an occupational accident) can make back pain particularly resistant to treatment, and an integrated approach to these aspects should be adopted.

---

[1]When we walk down a slope we assume a position of lumbar hyperlordosis to keep our balance. When we go up, we tend to flex our spine. Hyperlordosis reduces the diameter of the lumbar canal, exacerbating the symptoms…

TABLE 1.2 "Yellow flags" in low back pain, psychosocial criteria for a bad prognosis

Questions	Indicators of a bad prognosis
Previous sick leave for low back pain?	Yes
What do you think is causing the pain?	Focus on a structural cause Pessimistic or catastrophic attitude
What do you think can help you?	Nothing Others, doctors, but not the patient
How do others react to your pain?	They are hostile Over-protective
What do you do to make the pain bearable?	Passive attitudes: rest, escape, avoiding activities, etc.
Do you think you'll work again? When?	No, or don't know

These factors have been called "yellow flags" (Table 1.2).

The Regional Clinical Examination

A general rheumatologic examination gives us an immediate indication of the existence of pain or limited mobility in the lumbar spine. Pain that appears particularly during flexion suggests pathology of the disks or vertebral bodies. Pain that appears particularly during extension points to disease of the facet joints or spondylolisthesis.

Pain on all types of movement is an alarm signal.

if the patient complains of low back pain or the examination shows anomalies, we need to look into it further.

Inspection

Look at the curves of the spine when the patient is standing (Fig. 1.6). The lumbar spine normally shows mild physiological lordosis.

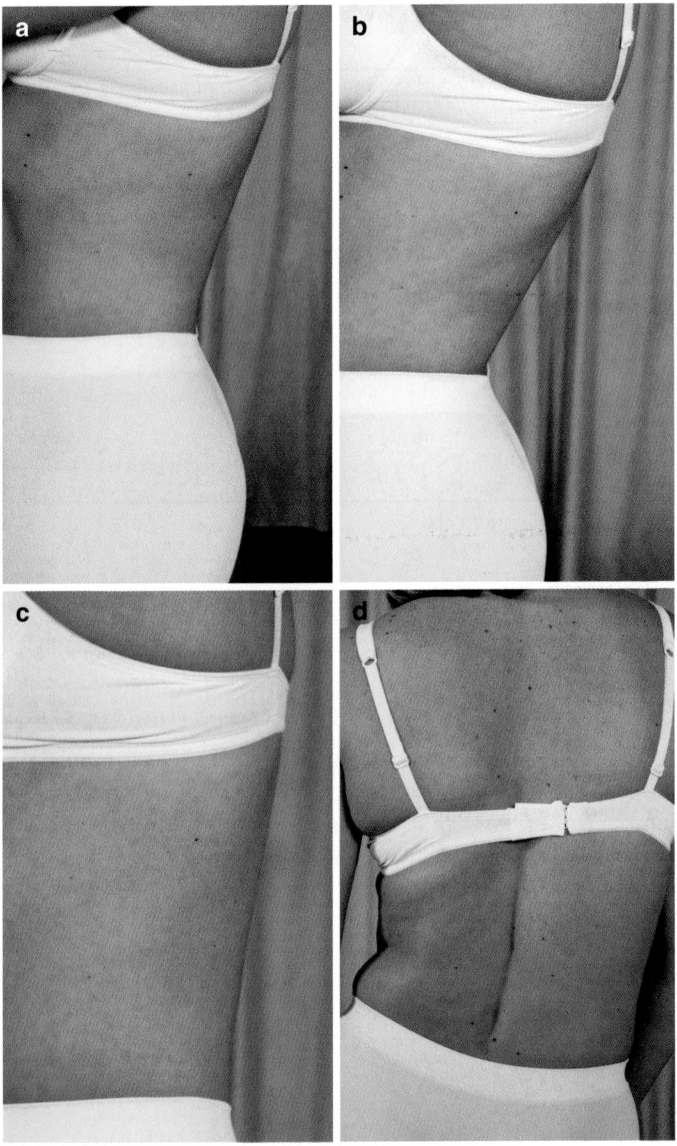

FIGURE 1.6 Normal and abnormal curves of the lumbar spine. (**a**) Normal. (**b**) Hyperlordosis. (**c**) Lost lumbar lordosis. (**d**) Scoliosis

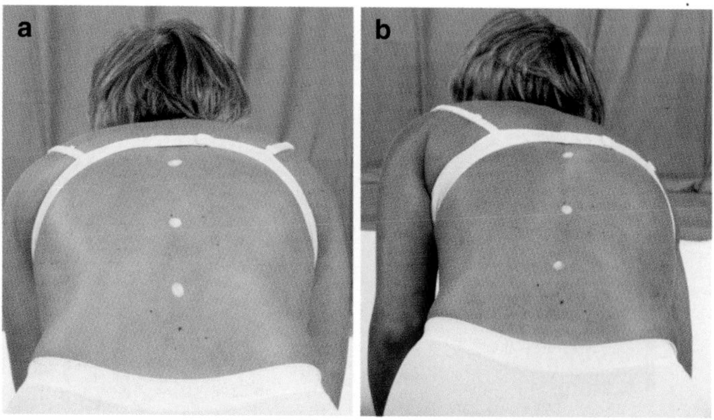

FIGURE 1.7 Postural scoliosis (**a**) is corrected by flexing the lumbar spine: the spinous processes are aligned and the shoulders level. In structural, fixed scoliosis (**b**), the abnormal curve persists in flexion and the shoulders and chest wall are assymetrical

Common, non-specific low back pain is often associated with an exaggeration of this curvature – hyperlordosis. This condition is more common in women and may be aggravated by wearing high heeled shoes and lack of muscle strength in the abdominal wall. Whatever the cause, hyperlordosis means that the spine's support structures are overloaded and, presumably, there are conflicts of space on the extension surface that lead to exacerbation and maintenance of the pain. One of the aims of treatment is to correct this.

Reduced lordosis or straightening of the lumbar spine is most commonly seen in advanced cases of ankylosing spondylitis.

Scoliosis is also a cause of pain. It may be merely postural or be caused by rotation of the vertebrae (congenital or acquired). If severe, structural scoliosis should be referred to a specialist.Postural scoliosis can normally be corrected by physiotherapy or by compensating for leg-length discrepancy. To distinguish between the two, we ask the standing patient to flex his spine completely and touch the floor with his fingers,keeping knees extended. Postural scoliosis is corrected in this position: the spine is aligned and the shoulders are at the same height. In fixed, structural scoliosis the deviation remains and the shoulders or thoracic wall are asymmetrical (Fig. 1.7).

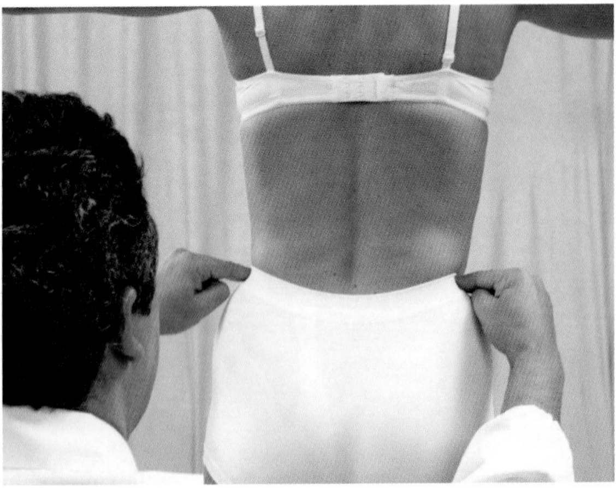

FIGURE 1.8 Clear identification of the iliac crests helps detection of lower limb length discrepancy, a common cause of scolliosis and low back pain

One of the most common causes of scoliosis and low back pain is leg-length discrepancy. This condition should be found during the clinical examination. While observing the patient from the back, with his knees extended, put your index fingers on theiliac crest on each side and evaluate their relative position (Fig. 1.8).

Scoliosis caused by leg-length discrepancy disappears when the patient is sitting. If we suspect significant discrepancy, a precise measurement of the lower limbs can be obtained with x-rays. Correction of significant differences (>1 cm) using insoles or built-up heels can relieve scoliosis, thus treating and preventing back pain.

Palpation

The joints in the spine are not accessible to direct palpation, as they are too deep.

With the patient lying face down, press the spinous processes from L1 to S2 with the tips of your fingers. Some

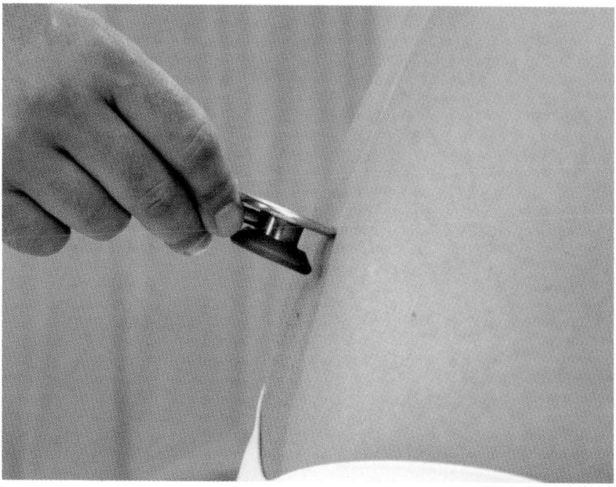

FIGURE 1.9 Exerting pressure between the spinous process with the stethoscope head will cause pain in interspinous ligamentitis

authors suggest percussion of the spine with a closed fist. Also palpate the paravertebral muscles on either side. Note the location of the pain. The more localized it is, the more relevant it is to the diagnosis.

if the pain is localized, try to distinguish between pain in the longitudinal ligaments (ligamentitis) and vertebral body pain. In the former case, the pain is more intense when you palpate between the spinous processes. This evaluation may be more reliable with the patient sitting with the lumbar spine flexed, using the edge of the chest piece of the stethoscope to palpate the ligaments between the processes (Fig. 1.9).

Mobilization

When the general rheumatologic examination shows limited mobility of the lumbar spine, it can be useful to quantify it more accurately, especially to assess the results of treatment at subsequent visits.

Lateral flexion of the lumbar spine can be quantified by measuring the distance between the tips of the fingers and

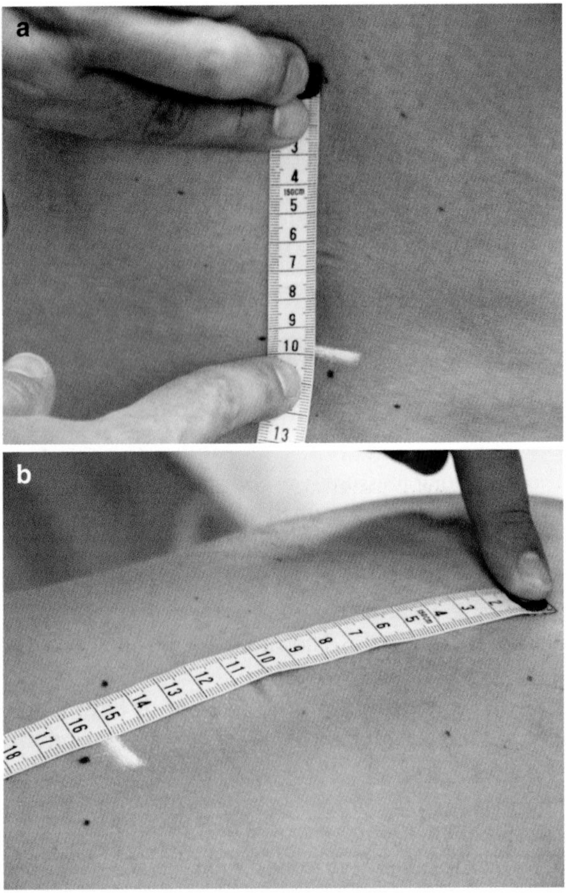

FIGURE 1.10 Schober's test: quantification of lumbar spine flexion. The lower reference is at the level of the iliac crests

the floor when the patient leans to one side and the other with his legs extended and his palm touching his leg.

The best way to quantify flexion is to use **Schober's test** (Fig. 1.10).

With the patient standing at ease, use a marker to indicate the spot where the line joining the iliac crests crosses the middle of the lumbar spine (L4–L5). Using a tape measure, make another mark 10 cm above this point. Ask the patient to flex his spine forward as far as possible and measure the distance between the two marks. In young, healthy individuals, the distance should now be more than 15 cm. Note that mobility of the spine diminishes naturally with age.

Examination of the Sacroiliac Joints

if the back pain is inflammatory, also palpate the sacroiliac joints with the patient lying face down (Fig. 1.11a). Then exert posteroanterior pressure on the median line of the sacrum to see if it causes sacroiliac pain (Fig. 1.11b). After this, ask the patient to lie on his back. Cross your arms and lean your hands on the anterior superior iliac spines (i.e. if you are facing the patient, your left hand on the patient's left anterior superior iliac spine and vice-versa. Push posterolaterally, springing the sacrum on and spread the patient's pelvis (Fig. 1.11c). The manoeuver is positive if it causes pain in the sacral region, suggesting compromise of the sacroiliac joints (the pain under your hands is not significant… but it can be particularly intense in patients with fibromyalgia).

When you have finished examining the abdomen and lower limbs, ask the patient to get up, raising his body without using the arms. The difficulty he experiences gives you an idea of the state of his abdominal muscles, which are the lumbar spine's best friends!

Neurological Examination

Any suggestion of neurogenic compromise should lead to a neurological examination of the lower limbs.

The distribution of the sensitive dermatomes of the lumbar roots is shown in Fig. 1.12 Table 1.3 shows the muscle strength corresponding to each root.

The patellar reflex depends on L3-L4 and the Achilles reflex on S1. Sciatic pain is caused by irritation of the roots of L5 and/or S1. It is characterized by its lumbar location with

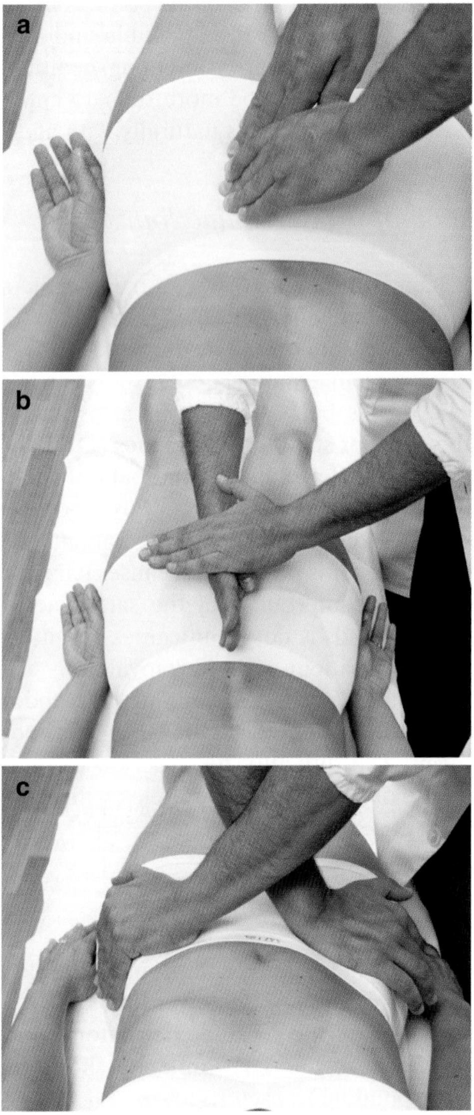
a
b
c

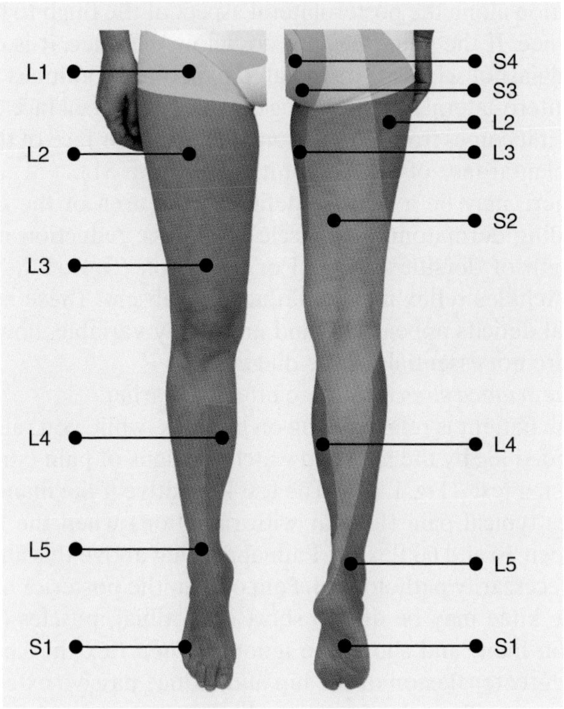

FIGURE 1.12 Skin dermatomes of lumbar nerve roots

TABLE 1.3 Radicular dependence of the strength in the lower limbs

	Anterior face	Posterior face
Hip	L2, L3 (flexion)	L4, L5 (extension)
Knee	L3, L4 (extension)	L5, S1 (flexion)
Foot	L4, L5 (dorsiflexion)	S1, S2 (extension)

FIGURE 1.11 Examining the sacroiliac joints. (**a**) Palpation. (**b**) Mobilization. With the patient lying face down, the sacrum is pressed anteriorly at midline, thus forcing the abduction of sacroiliac joints. (**c**) Mobilization. With the patient lying prone the observer tries to push the antero-superior iliac spines apart. The maneuvers are positive if they cause pain in the sacroiliac joints

radiation along the posterolateral aspect of the thigh to below the knee. If the pain does not go below the knee, it is called cruralgia, not sciatica. The radiated pain often continues along the antero-lateral face of the leg down to the dorsal face of the foot (if it comes from L5) or along the posterior face of the leg and plantar face of the foot (if it comes from S1).

There may be a sensory deficit in the area of the corresponding dermatome or muscle weakness: reduction of the strength of dorsiflexion (L5) or extension (S1) of the foot. The Achilles reflex may be reduced or absent. These neurological deficits appear late and are highly variable, however, and are not essential for the diagnosis.

The sciatica stretch tests are effective earlier.

The patient is relaxed lying on his back, while you raise his extended leg by the heel and watch for signs of pain (straight leg rising test – Fig. 1.13a). The test is positive if the maneuver causes typical pain (lumbar with radiation) when the hip is between 30 and 60 flexion. Pain appearing above this angle is not necessarily pathological. Pain only in the posterior aspect of the knee may be due to short ischiotibial muscles (common in men) and should be ignored. Then flex the knee to allow greater flexion of the hip and induce passive extension of the knee. Typical pain with radiation constitutes Las gue's sign (Fig. 1.13b).

The diagnosis of sciatica can be reinforced if Bragard's test elicits typical pain. The lower limb is passively elevated, with the knee extended, to the *maximum tolerated without pain.* The foot is then forced into dorsiflexion (Fig. 1.13c). If these signs are inconsistent, we should suspect anxiety or manipulation on the part of the patient or also pseudo-sciatica (due to piriform muscle syndrome or trochanteric bursitis, for example).[2]

---

[2]One way of distinguishing manipulation by the patient is to cause flexion of the leg with extension of the knee, while the patient is sitting. The manoeuver reproduces Lasègue's test, but is not so well known…

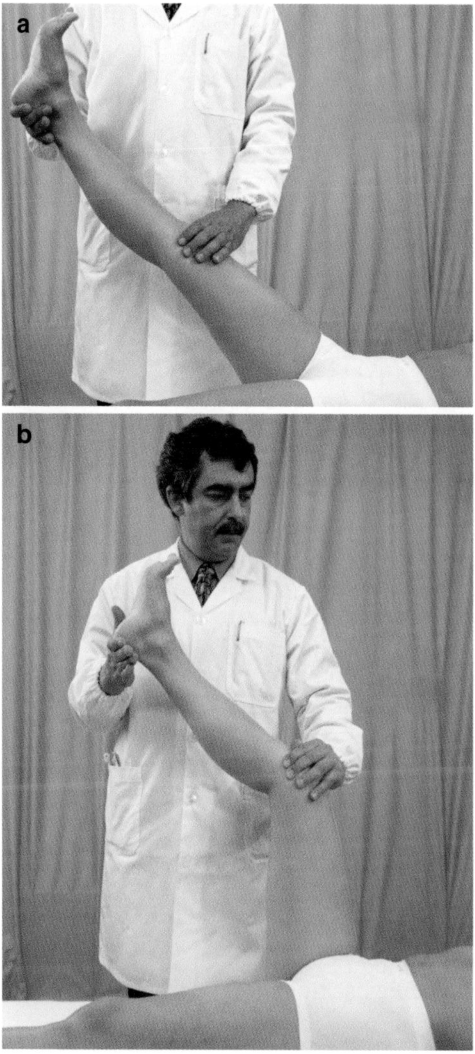

FIGURE 1.13 Sciatic nerve stretch tests. (**a**) Passive elevation of the lower limb, with knee extended. (**b**) Lasègue's test. (**c**) Bragard's test (Vd. text for explanations)

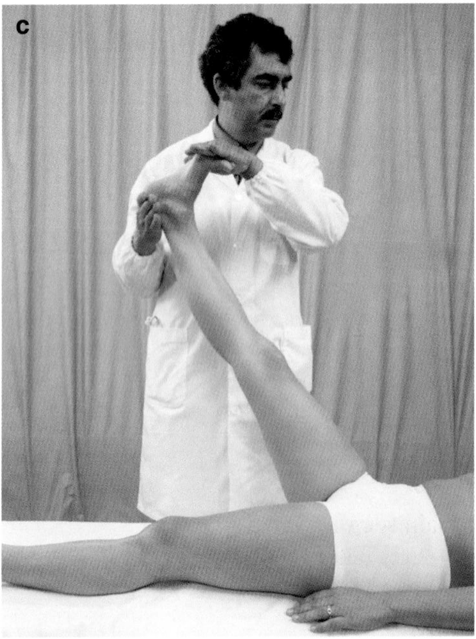

FIGURE 1.13 (continued)

After the enquiry and the clinical examination, the common causes of low back pain can be divided into five main clinical groups.

- Mechanical back pain
- Inflammatory back pain
- Neurogenic back pain
- Back pain of systemic origin
- Psychogenic back pain

Mechanical back pain
The pain is related to movement and exercise and is relieved by rest. Prolonged standing or sitting can exacerbate the pain. It does not get worse with Valsava's

maneuvers. The pain may radiate to the knee but not below it, and is not of a dysesthetic nature. There is no neurological deficit.

Spinal osteoarthritis, postural impairment and small muscle or ligament distensions are the most common underlying causes.

It represents about 90% of cases of back pain in ambulatory clinical practice today and is therefore extremely common.

Inflammatory back pain

The pain is worse at night and in the morning, and is accompanied by prolonged morning stiffness. Exercise relieves the pain.

Seronegative spondyloarthropathies are the most common cause but do not account for more than 1% of all back pain seen in general practice.

Neurogenic back pain

The pain is mechanical, but radiates to below the knee following a dermatome (usually L5 or S1). There is often paresthesia and the pain is exacerbated by Valsava's maneuvers. A neurological examination may find impaired strength, sensitivity and myotatic reflexes. Sciatic stretch tests are usually positive. Very occasionally, neurogenic back pain can begin in higher roots, with corresponding radiation and neurological examination results.

Herniated disks are the most common cause, but it may also be due to osteophytosis, fractures, neoplasm, etc.

Back pain of systemic orgin

The pain may have a varied rhythm but is not usually relieved by lying down. Clinical examination often reveals a clearly defined area of tenderness.

The pain may be referred from intra-abdominal viscera or reflect serious local bony or disc pathologies such as metastases or infection. Systemic manifestations like fever, weight loss or abdominal pain and onset before the age of 30 or after 50 should arouse suspicion.

Psychogenic back pain

Purely psychogenic low back pain is rare. Nevertheless, the patient may consciously or unconsciously exaggerate the manifestations of pain in situations such as depression, labor disputes, secondary gain or a manipulative personality.

A psychogenic component may naturally accompany clinical causes of pain and should be given due attention.

Our suspicions should be aroused when the description is particularly dramatic and colorful and the functional limitations described conflict too much with the physical examination of the patient. Multiple, spurious complaints, such as migratory paresthesia, a cold sensation in the back or intense pain on a superficial touch, are common and suggestive. The neurological examination is usually inconsistent.

Consider the possibility of fibromyalgia.

Typical Cases

1.A. Chronic Back Pain (I)

It was the third time that Manuel, a 68-year old pensioner, had come to emergency and always for the same reason: intense pain in the upper lumbar region that kept him awake at night. The pain was rather erratic: it never went away completely and was particularly intense early in the day, in the late morning and in the evening. He denied any local stiffness and insisted that the pain was not related to movement. There seemed to be some radiation to the abdomen.

In fact, the patient had been suffering from intermittent backache for many years but this was different. It used to be typically mechanical, related to exercise and went away completely on lying down. On his previous visits to emergency he had been given anti-inflammatories, which, according to the patient, seemed to exacerbate the pain. He denied any relevant systemic manifestations, other than slight weakness. He had a past medical history of "gastritis" and indigestion with no other relevant symptoms.

Examination of the spine showed slight limitation of flexion, without pain on local palpation or mobilization. Palpation of the abdomen elicited tenderness in the epigastric region, without guarding.

Consider the differential diagnosis…

Let us make a list of the dominant characteristics in this clinical condition:

- Chronic, mechanical low back pain that has changed recently
- An uncharacteristic rhythm but perhaps… peptic?
- A perfectly normal local examination
- Exacerbated by anti-inflammatories
- A history of gastritis

And… there is the possible diagnosis!

We decided to test the possibility before conducting an upper digestive endoscopy. We gave our patient 15 cc of antacid and… the pain soon got better.

An endoscopy the next day confirmed a perforated duodenal ulcer in the posterior wall, most likely causing irritation of the celiac plexus and lumbar pain.

Referred Back Pain

Main Points

This may appear at any age.

The pain is unrelated to movement.

The rhythm varies with the underlying disease.

An examination of the lumbar spine finds insufficient abnormalities to account for the pain.

The systematic enquiry and physical examination looking for visceral lesions that may lead to lumbar radiation are the key to the diagnosis.

Typical Cases

1.B. Acute Low Back Pain (I)

I went to see a friend at his home. I found him surrounded by cushions in his dressing gown on the couch, to which he had moved with difficulty after 3 days in bed with acute low back pain that had appeared when he was trying to lift a heavy object from his car. The pain radiated strongly down the posterolateral aspect of his left thigh and leg down to the plantar aspect of his foot, like an electric shock. It was exacerbated by any attempt at movement, leaving a persistent burning sensation along his lower limb. I asked him if the pain was worse when he coughed or sneezed. "Excruciating," he said. He had never felt such pain in all his 38 years.

He had already taken diclofenac (a fast-acting non-steroidal) and intramuscular injections of high doses of Vitamin B12. The relief he felt with the tablets lasted 3-4 hours. He was scheduled to have an MRI of his lumbar spine the following week.

On clinical examination I noted clear, painful limitation of flexion of the spine. There was a scoliotic deviation to the left with increased tension of the paravertebral muscles on the same side. Las gue's sign was positive on the left at about 50 flexion of the hip joint. His left ankle reflex was clearly reduced in comparison to the right. Muscle strength on extension of the left foot was diminished but there were no apparent changes in sensitivity to pain.

Summarize the patient's condition.[3]

What is your diagnosis?

Would you ask for any diagnostic tests? Would an MRI be of any use?

What would you advise the patient to do?

There could be no doubt that Alberto was suffering from sciatica. At his age, and in the absence of any previous pathology, he most likely had a herniated disk, with compression of the S1 root.

---

[3]Acute low back pain with sciatic radiation and neurological deficit in a young man.

I suggested that he began to take a full dose of anti-inflammatory to cover all 24 hours. I recommended additional medication with a muscle relaxant and a further analgesic, as needed. I said that he might find relief lying down, with his spine, hips and knees flexed. Hot baths might also be useful.

I recommended escalating gentle exercises for his lumbar spine spasm and suggested that he went back to his normal life as soon as possible. I saw no point in continuing the vitamins or having the MRI before seeing how his condition progressed. I did not arrange any diagnostic tests.

My friend went back to work after 3 days and discontinued all treatment after about a week. I strongly urged him to do regular exercises with particular attention to his lumbar and abdominal muscles. I advised him to lose some weight and gave him some advice about posture to protect the lumbar region.

Sciatica

Main Points

Diagnosing sciatica involves:

- Lumbar pain radiating to below the knee with or without paresthesia
- Positive sciatica stretch tests
- Neurological deficit (inconstant)

It appears mainly in young people in association with a herniated disk or spondylolisthesis and, more rarely, in the elderly (compression due to osteophytes or expansive lesion – neoplasm?)

When it is typical, no diagnostic tests are necessary. Initial treatment consists of short-term rest, analgesics and muscle relaxants.[4]

[4]Around the compressed root, there is always some inflammatory reaction that exacerbates and perpetuates the pain. The fullest possible analgesia is important to prevent the vicious circle of pain and muscle spasm that plays an important role in these situations. Early, gentle exercise is important in facilitating the withdrawal of the herniated core. Regular, long-term exercise and care with posture are essential in preventing recurrences.

The patient should be encouraged to resume normal physical activity as soon as possible and to take regular exercise for the spine.

If the pain and neurological deficit persist after four to eight weeks of conservative treatment, it is worth considering physical therapy or even surgery.

Typical Cases

1.C. Chronic Back Pain (II)

Aurora, a 68-year old patient, had been suffering from low back pain for over four years. At first, the pain was recurrent with pain-free periods in between episodes but it got progressively more intense and continuous, forcing her to go to her doctor again. Recently, the pain was located diffusely in the lumbar region. When asked about radiated pain, she said that her buttocks and thighs sometimes hurt too. She had not noticed any paresthesia, but she felt some "weakness" in her legs. The pain was exacerbated by walking and the little exercise that she was still able to take. It was relieved by lying flat on her back.

She also described mechanical pain in both knees, especially when going up and down stairs.

She had had non-insulin-dependent diabetes for about 10 years and was taking medication for hypertension and cardiac insufficiency. She denied any recent weight loss (the opposite…) and had not noticed any changes in her digestive or intestinal habits, or in the appearance of her stools or urine.

Our clinical examination showed an obese woman (weighing 84.2 kg and 1.51 m tall) with difficulty walking. Examination of her chest, abdomen and breasts was normal. The lumbar curvature of her spine was highly accentuated, but without scoliosis. The iliac crests were symmetrical. Active mobilization of the cervical and lumbar spine was painfully limited, especially in extension. There was patellofemoral crepitus, but no other anomalies in the examination of her legs.

Palpation of the lumbar spine and the paravertebral muscles was diffusely painful. A summary neurological examination showed no loss of muscle strength. There were absent ankle reflexes bilaterally. There was a symmetrical loss of sensitivity to pain in her lower legs and feet. The patient was unable to get up from the examining table without supporting herself on her arms, even when starting from 45 flexion.

What is the most probable diagnosis?

What tests and treatment would you suggest?

We decided that this was a case of chronic, non-specific mechanical back pain. The patient's age and pain on extension made it likely that she was suffering from Spinal osteoarthritis. This would not affect the treatment, however, so we did not request any imaging. The reduced ankle reflexes and the apparent loss of distal sensitivity were probably related to her diabetes mellitus.

Her obesity, hyperlordosis and weakness of the abdominal muscles were exacerbating factors, justifying specific intervention.

We explained the situation to our patient, stressing the effect of her obesity both on the pain and on the diabetes. She was strongly advised to go on a low calorie diet. We reassured the patient as to the likely prognosis of backache, emphasizing the need to stay active and do regular exercises at home to strengthen the spinal and abdominal muscles. We gave her a leaflet of low back exercises and advice as to the best way to protect her back: the right footwear, a firm mattress, how to pick up heavy items, etc.

We prescribed a simple analgesic to be taken as required and arranged to see her again in about two months, hoping to find her thinner and more energetic…

We have indicated some extra-articular characteristics for this patient. Could any of them have an impact on the way we examined and treated her?[5]

Common Chronic Back Pain

Main Points

This is a very common condition in clinical practice, especially in the elderly.

It is defined as lumbar pain lasting more than six months with no specific diagnosis.

This diagnosis requires the exclusion of any suggestions of specific pathology ("red flags"). The pain is mechanical, with periods of exacerbation and relief. It often radiates to the buttocks. A local examination may show reduced mobility, especially in flexion and extension. Palpation is diffusely painful. The neurological examination is normal.

It is often associated with depression, postural deficiency and occupational factors. No additional diagnostic tests are necessary.

Treatment focuses on mobility and not the pain: analgesia, appropriate regular physical exercise, advice on posture, reaching ideal weight and continuing normal physical activity.

Typical Cases

1.D. Acute Back Pain (II)

Jorge Esteves, a generally healthy office worker aged 36, went to the emergency department because of acute-onset back pain after heavy lifting when moving house.

[5]Yes. Hypertension and heart failure can be aggravated by non-steroidal anti-inflammatories which can also result in edema and nitrogen retention. The diabetes would contraindicate the use of corticosteroids, if any other situation made them necessary. Type II diabetes and obesity reduce the risk of osteoporosis, which we should always consider in a patient aged 68.

The pain radiated to the buttocks and the posterior aspect of the thigh, but not lower. It was exacerbated by any attempt at movement and by coughing and sneezing. Clinical examination showed scoliosis concave to the left, with obvious contracture of the left paravertebral muscles. Movements of the spine were painful in all directions. The summary neurological examination was normal. Sciatica stretching tests exacerbated the lumbar pain, with no typical radiation.

What would you do in this situation?

We assured the patient and his wife that there was nothing seriously wrong with him and that the pain would go away in one or two weeks. We recommended rest for only a day or two and suggested that he gradually went back to his daily routine as soon as possible, even if he still had some pain. We prescribed paracetamol (1 g, four times a day) and a muscle relaxant (for 1 week) and suggested hot baths for relaxation. We gave him advice on posture and a regular exercise plan, which he should start after the acute episode had resolved.

Acute, Mechanical Back Pain

Main Points

It occurs frequently in young individuals, generally associated with lifting.

Muscle contracture, frequently obvious on palpation, plays a decisive role in the initiation and continuation of the process.

In the absence of any unusual clinical elements, no diagnostic tests are necessary.

Treatment is designed to relieve the pain and enable the patient to resume normal physical activity as soon as possible.

Prolonged rest is counterproductive as it facilitates progression to chronicity.

Manipulation of the lumbar spine by an experienced practitioner may be useful in the first four weeks of pain.

Most cases resolve in four to eight weeks. If pain persists for longer the patient should be reassessed or sent to a specialist.

It is important to reassure the patient, and initiate a long-term plan for protecting the joints.

Typical Cases

1.E. Chronic Back Pain (III)

Francisco Garção, a 58-year old farmer, was referred urgently to our department because of low back pain with some unusual characteristics. The pain was unrelated to movement and was more intense at night. It had originally been related to farm work but was not relieved by rest or anti-inflammatories. His doctor requested some tests, which showed some surprising alterations. Although the spinal x-ray suggested osteoarthritis in L4–L5, his ESR was elevated (45 mm in the first hour).

Does this seem like ordinary low back pain? Why?
What additional information would you try to get?

When we examined this patient, we were able to confirm the information obtained from his referral letter. Systematic enquiry revealed that he had had a feeling of fever for a few months. He had also noted some weight loss (about 5 kg in the last 3 months). His work involved frequent contact with goats and he regularly drank goat's milk.

The pain was clearly located over L4–L5. Our summary neurological examination was normal.

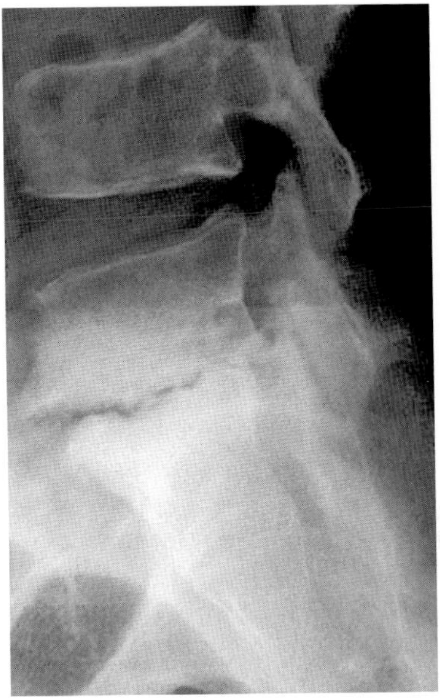

FIGURE 1.14 Lateral spine X-ray of the patient described in clinical case "Chronic low back pain (III)." There is loss of disk height, irregularity and sclerosis of vertebral endplates. An anterior osteophyte in L5 demonstrates associated osteoarthritis

What possible diagnoses are there?

What diagnostic tests might be useful?

The x-ray was clearly compatible with discitis (Fig. 1.14). A CT-guided biopsy produced material from which mycobacterium tuberculosis was identified.

The patient underwent prolonged treatment which resulted in clinical improvement and normalization of the lab results. However, he still has persistent mechanical low back pain.

Spondylodiscitis

Main Points

Discitis (vertebral disk infection) is relatively rare but constitutes a rheumatologic emergency.

It requires rapid diagnosis and treatment to avoid the risk of irreversible neurological sequelae. On suspicion of this disease, the patient should be referred to a specialist immediately without waiting for any radiological alterations, which appear late.

Note the inflammatory rhythm of the pain, its precise location and any association with systemic symptoms of infection.

The acute-phase reactants are high and aid diagnosis and follow-up of treatment.

Staphylococcus aureus, streptococci, Mycobacterium tuberculosis and Brucella mellitensis, are the agents most commonly involved.

In later stages, a plain film of the spine shows loss of intervertebral space and lack of definition of the vertebral endplates sometimes with erosions. The picture may, however, be indistinguishable from ordinary spondyloarthropathy.

It is essential to conduct a biopsy for culture and antibiotic sensivities.

Typical Cases

1.F. Chronic Back Pain (IV)

Carlos, a 21-year old student and a keen amateur cyclist, came to us because of low back pain that had been developing for about two years. At the beginning, the pain was occasional and related to long periods studying at his desk or with more intensive sport. More recently, however, he noticed that the pain was becoming more persistent and was particularly severe in the morning, associated with stiffness.

The pain would sometimes wake him up at night. It also got worse after sitting for a long time, but was relieved by exercising the spine.

The pain affected the lower lumbar region and radiated to both buttocks, but no lower. He denied any clinical manifestations of the skin, mucosa or digestive tract.

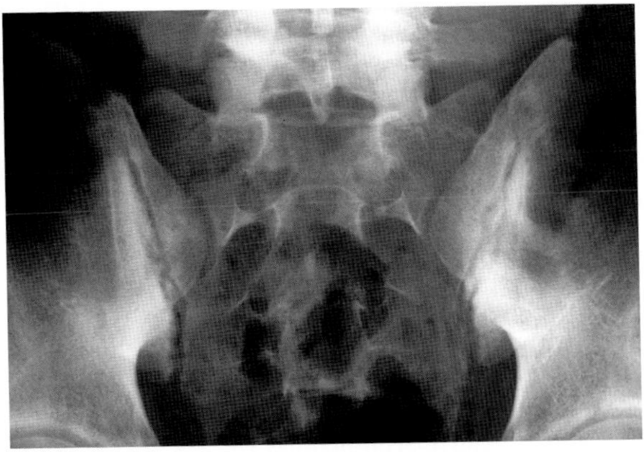

FIGURE 1.15 Anterior view of the lumbar spine. Clinical case "Chronic low back pain (IV)." Note the bone sclerosis surrounding the sacroiliac joints associated with blurring and erosions of the joint margins: bilateral sacroiliítis

Are there any alarm signals in this enquiry?

What are the potentially most important aspects of the physical examination?

Mobility of the spine was painless but slightly reduced (Schober 10-13.8 cm). Assessment of the sacroiliac joints was positive, causing pain in the lumbosacral region. No abnormalities were founding in the skin.

Summarize this clinical condition.[6]

Consider the most probable diagnoses and the diagnostic tests required.

The clinical information provided pointed strongly to the possibility of ankylosing spondylitis. This diagnosis was confirmed by an x-ray of the pelvis which showed typical changes in both sacroiliac joints (Fig. 1.15). The hemoglobin and ESR were normal.

[6]Inflammatory lumbosacral pain in a young man with no systemic manifestations. Probable sacroiliitis.

What treatment would you prescribe?

We began therapy with non-steroidal anti-inflammatories. We explained the nature of the condition and its foreseeable development to the patient, taking an optimistic attitude about his prognosis. We particularly stressed his own role in the treatment: care with posture, regular flexibility exercises for the lumbar spine, breathing exercises, giving up smoking, watching for side effects of the medications, and regular medical checkups. We suggested that he might want to join the Association of Patients with Ankylosing Spondylitis.

Seronegative Spondyloarthropathies

Main Points

The inflammatory rhythm is an important alarm signal in low back pain - it always warrants careful attention.

Ankylosing spondylitis is the most common of the seronegative spondyloarthropathies (types of arthritis classified together because of their tendency to involve the axial skeleton).

Males are more commonly affected and the manifestations normally begin in their late teens or twenties.

A careful examination of the sacroiliac joints with specific maneuvers is crucial in identifying sacroiliitis.

The systematic enquiry is important in identifying features associated with the different diseases: psoriasis, urethritis, conjunctivitis, diarrhea, etc…

Radiological alterations appear relatively late, but confirm the diagnosis.

Typical Cases

1.G. Acute Back Pain (III)

Celeste Craveiro, a 67-year old housewife, came to the emergency department with severe thoracic and lumbar pain that had appeared the day before following a minor fall at home, with no other consequences. The pain was continuous, only slightly relieved by rest and exacerbated by all movements, including taking deep breaths.

She described occasional chronic low back pain for more than seven years, which responded to analgesics, though it had never been as intense as now. She had been monitored by her family doctor in a remote village for about 10 years for inflammatory joint pain in her hands, wrists, shoulders and feet. She was taking non-steroidals regularly and was given injections during flare-ups. Although she did not know the name of the injections, she said their effect was "miraculous" for 2-3 months. She described considerable difficulty in walking and was practically housebound. She had had a spontaneous menopause at the age of 48 and had been diabetic for three years. She denied any other symptoms in the systematic enquiry.

She's your patient! Is this common low back pain? Why? What possible diagnoses can you think of? How would you investigate them?

Our examination showed a frail patient, with hand deformities typical of rheumatoid arthritis: ulnar deviation of the fingers and swan-neck defor- mations. The skin of her hands was atrophic with some hemorrhagic suffusion. She had slight Cushingoid facies and a buffalo neck.

An examination of her spine showed accentuated thoracic kyphosis. Mobilization of the thoraco-lumbar spine was extremely painful in all directions. Palpation caused pain at the thoracolumbar junction.

A lateral x-ray of her thoracic and lumbar spines showed accentuated thoracic kyphosis with generalized radiological osteopenia and wedge- shaped deformation of the T12 and L1 vertebral bodies (Fig. 1.16).

A radioisotope bone scan showed that these fractures were recent. Her ESR was elevated, but the protein electrophoretic strip was normal.

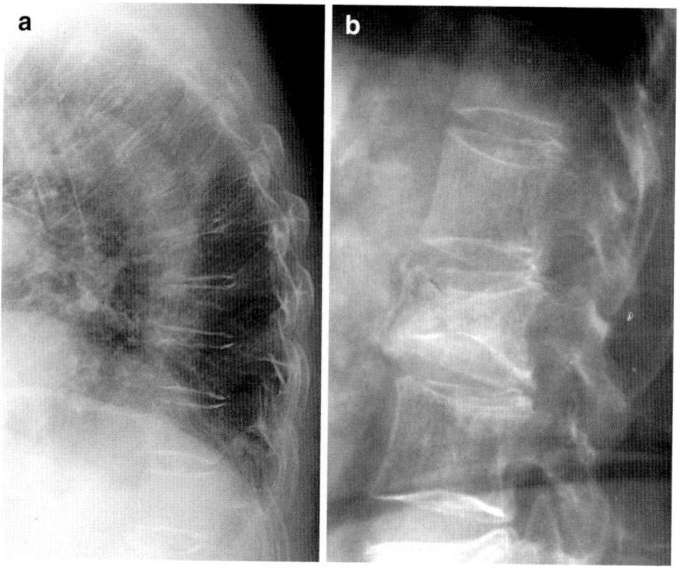

FIGURE 1.16 Clinical case "Acute low back pain (III)." (**a**) Compression deformity of L2 and radiological osteopenia of the dorsal and lumbar spine. (**b**) Osteoporotic fractures

What is your final diagnosis?
How would you treat it?

The patient was hospitalized for treatment of the acute episode and the introduction of appropriate therapy for her rheumatoid arthritis and osteoporosis.

Now think a little:

- What risk factors for osteoporosis could we identify in this patient?
- What signs of iatrogenic hypercortisolism did this patient have?
- How important is the protein strip is this context?[7]

---

[7]Signs: dorsal kyphosis, Cushingoid facies, cutaneous atrophy, diabetes, hypertension. Protein strip: in a patient of this age, with bone pain associated with severe osteoporosis, the possibility of multiple myeloma requires appropriate studies.

Osteoporotic Fracture

Main Points

This is a common situation in the elderly, especially women.

Although most osteoporotic vertebral fractures are progressive and clinically silent, they can cause acute, intense, incapacitating pain.

Osteoporotic vertebral fractures may occur spontaneously or as the result of a minor trauma. Symptomatic osteoporotic vertebral fracture requires urgent treatment and often hospitalization.

An osteoporotic fracture indicates a very high risk of further fractures and requires aggressive treatment of the osteoporosis.

Always assess the patient's risk factors for osteoporosis or signs suggesting its existence thus ensuring appropriate treatment.

Prolonged treatment with corticosteroids must always be associated with osteoporosis prophylaxis.

Typical Case

1.H. Acute Back Pain (IV)

Irene was clearly an obese, highly anxious patient who repeatedly described her pain in dramatic terms ("horrible, ghastly…"), making it difficult to focus our enquiry. Her history seemed to be dominated by pain located in the buttocks and radiating down the outer face of the left thigh and lower leg as far as her foot. The pain had started insidiously three months before. It was exacerbated by a variety of movements, but persisted at night, especially when lying on her left side. Valsava's maneuvers did not exacerbate the pain. She denied any paraesthesia, but felt that she "had no strength at all" in her left leg. The pain had been not been relieved by anti-inflammatory or other analgesic medication, or a course of physiotherapy with application of heat and mobilization of the lumbar spine.

Although our systematic enquiry abounded with all kinds of complaints it was inconsistent.

Are there any alarm signals?
Into what type of low back pain does this condition fit?
What aspects of the clinical examination would you focus on most?

Walking was difficult, with manifestations of pain at each step. Flexion of the spine triggered pain in the left hip, thigh and lower leg but was not limited. Palpation of the lumbar spine was diffusely painful. The sciatica stretch tests were contradictory and difficult to interpret: elevation of the limb caused pain at about 80 flexion of the hip. Lasé gue and Bragard triggered pain in the calves but not the spine. Her ankle reflexes were normal. Sensitivity to pain seemed intact. The strength of extension of the feet seemed reduced on the left side but the patient was able to walk on tiptoe.

Examination of the hip and knees showed no abnormalities, but deep palpation of the left greater trochanter was extremely painful and, according to the patient, reproduced the characteristics of the spontaneous pain.

What is your diagnosis?
What would you suggest to the patient?

We administered an injection of local anesthetic and corticosteroid into the painful points around the trochanter. Two minutes later the pain was less intense and the patient was able to make previously "impossible" movements.

Our diagnosis was trochanteric bursitis. We suggested bed rest for 24 hours and prescribed a topical anti-inflammatory to be massaged in lightly after the application of heat. We saw the patient again 2 weeks later and she was practically asymptomatic. We stressed the need to lose weight and take regular exercise.

Pseudo-Sciatica
Main Points
There are a number of situations that can simulate sciatica:
- Trochanteric bursitis;
- Piriform muscle syndrome;
- Iliotibial fascia syndrome.

The clinical examination suggests sciatica but the pain is not normally exacerbated by Valsava's maneuvers.

The neurological examination is negative or inconsistent.

Specific maneuvers for alternative causes in the physical examination are the key to the diagnosis.

Special Situations

Spinal Osteoarthritis

This is osteoarthritis of the joints in the spinal column, involving the intervertebral joints, the facet joints or both.

It is one of the most common findings on plain spine radiographs of patients with (and without!!) low back pain and is almost universal after the age of 55–60, although to varying degrees.

The radiograph may show osteophytes, which are sometimes large, with a reduction in the articular space and subchondral sclerosis (Fig. 1.17). The osteophytes of the facet joints may narrow the intervertebral foraminae leading to nerve root compression. The same is true for intervertebral osteophytes in a posterolateral location. The most obvious osteophytes in a standard film, however (marginal anterior and lateral), cannot cause nerve compression and are important mainly as indicators of general alterations in the morphology and function of the spine and not as individual sources of symptoms.

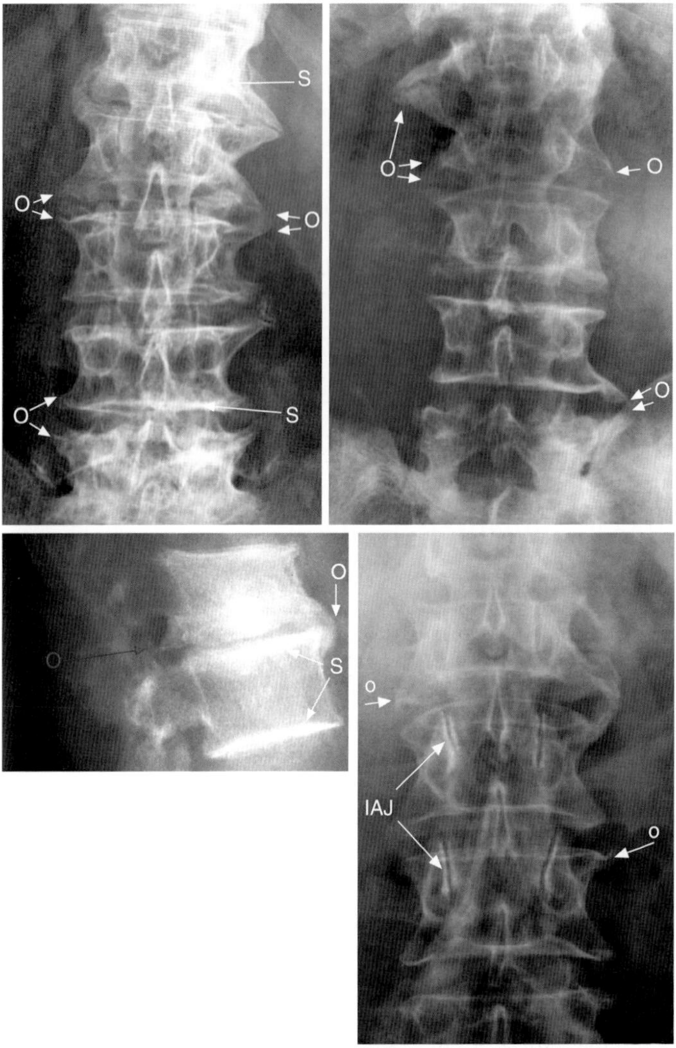

FIGURE 1.17 Osteoarthritis of the spine. *O* Osteophytes. Osteophytes projecting from the anterolateral aspect of the vertebral body can induce nerve root compression (red). *S* Subchondral sclerosis. *IAJ* Interapophyseal joints – can be visible in the antero-posterior radiograph and show signs of osteoarthritis

The radiological appearance of spinal osteoarthritis may easily lead us to attribute the symptoms to it. We should, however, bear two basic aspects in mind:

1. The correlation between the radiological appearance and clinical signs and symptoms is very poor. We are just as likely to examine patients with few or no symptoms and a "disastrous" plain film or to come up against just the opposite. The severity of the situation dep ends on the symptoms, not on the x-ray.
2. Spinal osteoarthritis only justifies specific treatment in exceptional cases (if there is a neurological deficit). Even in these cases, we have to give this care- ful thought as it requires surgery, which is not always successful. In most patients with low back pain and spinal osteo arthritis the treatment is the same as for other chronic mechanical low back pain without radiological alterations: focusing on mobility and not on the pain, on the patient's quality of life and not on his or her x-ray, and essentially aiming at relieving the symptoms and protecting the joints (exercise and keeping up normal physical activity).

Note That

Spinal Osteoarthritis:

- The correlation between the clinical examination and the x-ray is very poor.
- Specific treatment is only justified if there is neurological deficit or untreatable pain.
- For practical purposes it should not be considered a specific diagnosis. The clinical examination is decisive. Assessment and treatment follow the same principles for any kind of mechanical low back pain.

Diffuse Idiopathic Skeletal Hyperostosis

Diffuse idiopathic skeletal hyperostosis (DISH), also called Forrestier's disease, is a common condition and may be

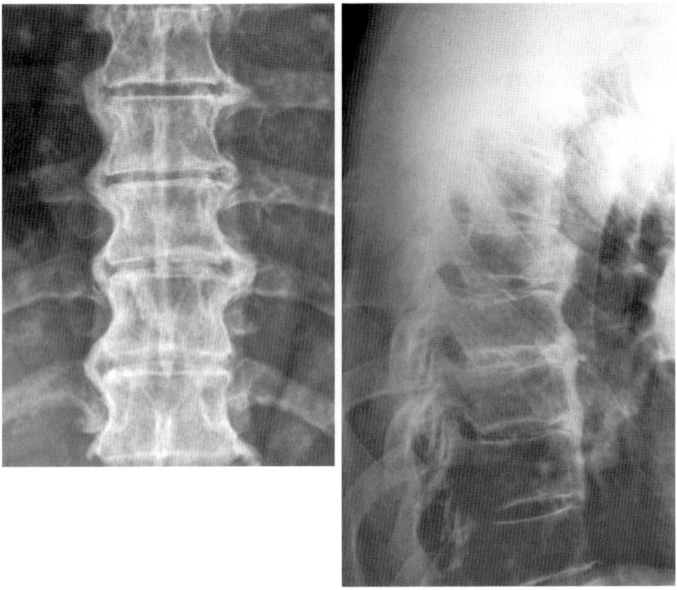

FIGURE 1.18 Diffuse Idiopathic Skeletal Hyperostosis (DISH). "Bone bridges" between adjacent vertebral bodies may suggest osteophytes but the disk space is preserved. Abnormalities frequently predominate on the right side of the body

mistaken for spinal osteoarthritis or ankylosing spondylitis in clinical or radiological examinations.

This disease involves calcification of the intervertebral ligaments, forming bony bridges between adjacent vertebrae and limiting their mobility. The calcifications form excrescences between adjacent vertebral bodies, usually predominating on the right side of the thoracic spine. A profile x-ray often shows calcification of the anterior vertebral ligament, in front of the anterior face of the vertebral body and intervertebral disks. To satisfy the radiological criteria of the disease at least four adjacent vertebral bodies must be involved.

Unlike spinal osteoar thritis, the height of the disk spaces is unchanged and there is no subchondral sclerosis (Fig. 1.18).

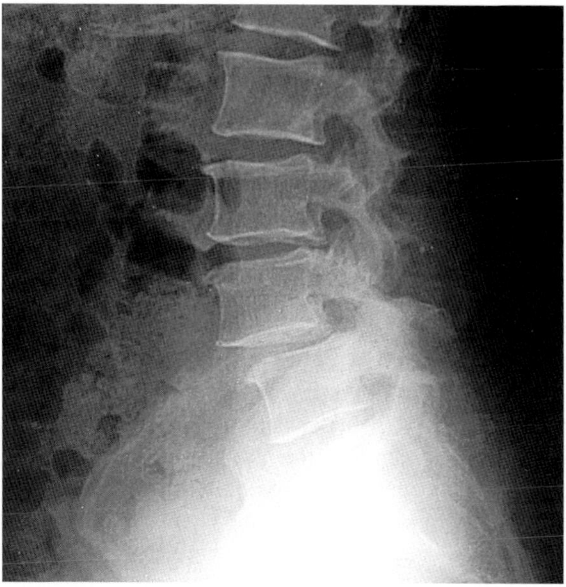

FIGURE 1.19 Spondylolisthesis. Anterior dislocation of one vertebral body over the underlying one

It is most common in middle-aged and elderly men and the statistics associate the risk with alcoholism and diabetes mellitus. The symptoms are few, usually limited to mechanical axial discomfort and reduced mobility.

Peripheral joints may be involved in this hyperostotic tendency, leading to early osteoarthritis with exuberant osteophytosis and often calcification of periarticular ligaments and entheses.

Treatment is essentially symptomatic.

Spondylolisthesis

This is caused by a defect in the vertebral isthmuses allowing the vertebral body to lose the fixation represented by the facet joints and slide over the underlying vertebra (Fig. 1.19). It is often congenital, but may be caused by trauma.

The relationship with clinical manifestations is highly variable. The patient may mention lumbar pain that is generally worse in extension. The greater the degree of dislocation, the greater the probability of its causing symptoms. On rare occasions it may cause nerve compression.

Treatment is essentially conservative (exercise, posture, reassurance), resorting to surgical stabilization in cases of severe symptoms.

Spina Bifida

This is caused by a congenital defect in the development of the lumbar spine, which consists of the duplication of the spinous processes, leaving the posterior wall of the spinal canal without complete coverage by bone.

It is very common and is a frequently reported radiological finding. In most cases, it is benign and asymptomatic, and should not normally be considered the cause of painful or neurogenic symptoms.

Fibromyalgia

Although the typical symptom of fibromyalgia is generalized pain, many patients with this condition locate the pain predominantly in the lumbar region. If the patient is not questioned carefully, we may focus our attention on this region and the underlying diagnosis is missed and thus the appropriate treatment not offered.

Diagnostic Tests

A common mistake in clinical practice is to request too many tests in cases of low back pain.

Most cases of low back pain are mechanical, with no alarm signals, and do not require any tests, as the clinical examination provides enough information to diagnose and treat it.

If we request spine radiographs for all these patients, we will find some kind of structural abnormality in many of them, especially varying degrees of spinal osteoarthritis. These findings should not, however, change our choice of treatment, as we do not have specific measures for each condition and the relationship between radiology and clinical examination is very weak. An investigation that does not change treatment is unnecessary!

In addition, unnecessary x-rays are far from harmless. The dose of radiation in repeated x-rays is by no means negligible, but the most important thing is the impact that these investigations and their findings have on the patients' approach to their condition. When faced with a structural diagnosis that they find hard to interpret, patients naturally focus on the disease and not on their mobility. This may reinforce their tendency to avoid exercise, which is the opposite of what is required, and also to justify their "role as a patient" or secondary gains.

If we want the patient to remain active in spite of the pain, it is better to play down irrelevant x-ray results than to lend them too much importance.

Diagnostic tests should depend on the clinical types of low back pain described above:

Mechanical Low Back Pain

In most cases no diagnostic tests are justified. If they are necessary to reassure an overanxious patient, we should limit them to the essential and avoid repeating them. The focus should remain on mobility and not on the pain or its cause.

Inflammatory Low Back Pain

As ankylosing spondylitis is the most common cause of this condition, it is worth requesting a anteroposterior x-ray of the pelvis to study the sacroiliac joints and two x-ray projections of the lumbar spine to look at vertebral morphology and detect any syndesmophytes. These plain films are also appropriate for other types of seronegative spondyloarthropathy. The abnormal findings are, however, relatively late and their absence should not rule out a clinically grounded diagnosis.

Neurogenic Low Back Pain

Clinical history and the physical examination are the basis of diagnosis. Electrophysiological studies may be warranted when we are in doubt as to neurological function. An ordinary x-ray of the spine in no way confirms or rules out radicular compression or its location. It may be useful only to ascertain the general state of the spine and the advisability of surgery.

CT or MRI scans are only justified if surgery is being considered. Otherwise, they can bring more problems than solutions. For example, MRI scans identify small disk anomalies in a large percentage of totally asymptomatic people. They can only be interpreted in the light of a clearly defined neurological deficit.

Low Back Pain of Systemic Origin

Tests will depend on the nature of our clinical suspicion (metastases, local infection or osteoporotic fracture), and can include a wide range of diagnostic studies: full blood count, acute phase reactants, plain films, bacteriological tests, biopsy, gastro-intestinal endoscopy, bone scintigraphy (metastases), densitometry, etc.

Psychogenic Low Back Pain

This is the situation in which unnecessary tests pose the greatest iatrogenic risk. Once we are sure of our diagnosis, we should be firm in establishing the limits to further investigations and in defending a clear, consistent plan of action.

Treatment

The treatment of low back pain with a specific diagnosis has already been addressed or will be dealt with in the appropriate chapters.

The comments below focus on the treatment of the most common condition, mechanical low back pain.

1. Educating the patient and preventing recurrences and chronicity

This is a fundamental aspect in treating low back pain.

We must first be aware of the patients' psychological relationship with their illness, encouraging them and their families to take a positive, proactive attitude in which the patients try to lead as full and normal a life as possible in spite of the pain. Overprotective attitudes, despondency and dependence on others should be fought. Optimism and self-sufficiency above all else!

The quality of the doctor-patient relationship has been scientifically identified as one of the most important factors in the progression of low back pain.

2. Rest and exercise

Contrary to traditional belief, it has been shown that prolonged rest actually extends the duration of acute low back pain episodes and promotes progression to chronicity. In acute, incapacitating low back pain the patient should be advised to rest for a short time (no more than 48-72 hours) and encouraged to return to normal life as soon as possible. Physiotherapy may be necessary in some cases.

We should make sufferers from chronic low back pain aware of the crucial importance of regular exercise and care with posture, if possible giving them leaflets like that shown in Fig. 1.20. These exercises are also the best way of preventing the recurrence of acute episodes.

We should also explain the importance of body weight and the best way of protecting the spine during daily activities as this helps the patient to adhere to the treatment. Patients must be made to feel that they play the most important role in their own treatment.

LOW BACK PAIN. Prescription of exercises.

Perform these exercises in the morning and in the evening. Start by repeating each exercise three times in each session and increase the number until you do them ten times per session, twice a day. Control your breathing. Perform the exercises as vigorously as possible, as long as you feel no pain after the exercise or in the following day.

Do exercise regularly: if you stop when the pain improves, it will most probably come back!

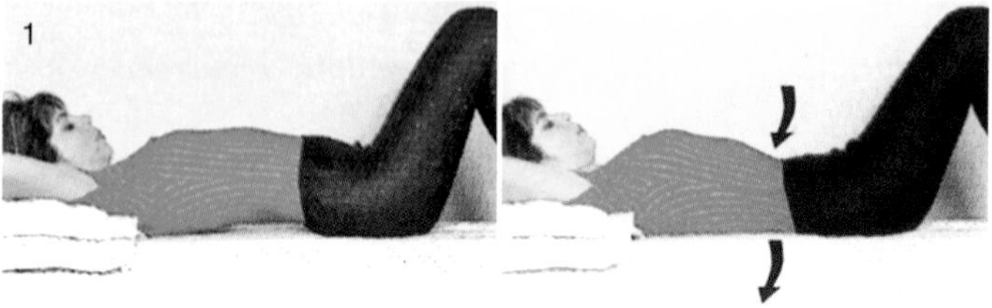

1. Mobilizing the spine. Lie on your back, on the bed or the floor, with knees bent and hands behind your head. Contract your tummy muscles and push your low back against the mattress. Count up to five and rest. Repeat.

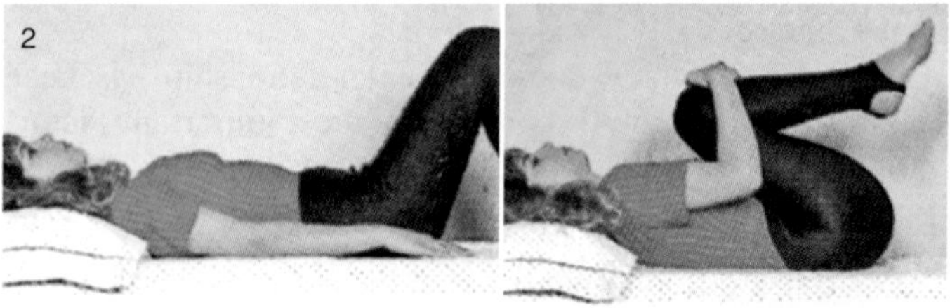

2. Bending the spine. Lie on your back on the bed. Hold your knees with your hands and pull them towards your chest as much as possible. Count up to five and rest. Repeat.

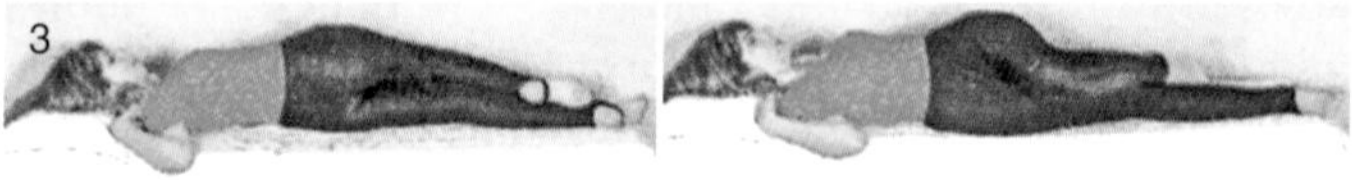

3. Turning the spine. While lying on your back, bend your right knee and move it over the left one, as far as possible, while keeping your shoulders in contact with the mattress or the floor. Count up to three and rest. Do the corresponding exercise with the left knee. Repeat.

FIGURE 1.20 Exercises for low back pain patients. Example of a patient leaflet. We suggest that the proposal is presented as a formal "prescription" (Produced in cooperation with Prof. J. Pascoa Pinheiro)

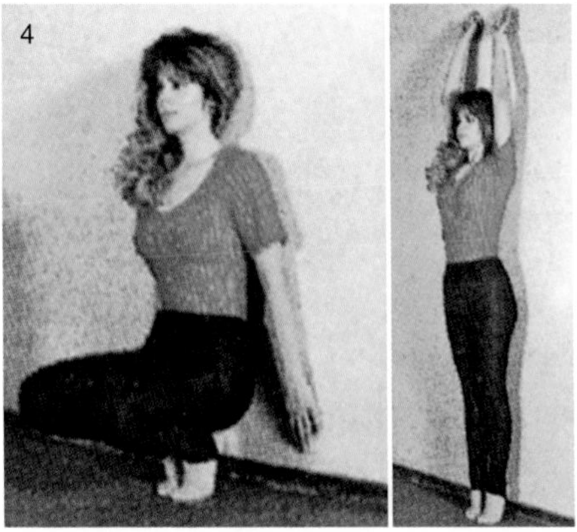

4. Stretching. Try to stretch your body as much as possible. Force your heels, buttocks, shoulders and back of the head against the wall. Bend your knees and stand again, reaching as high as possible, while keeping in touch with the wall.

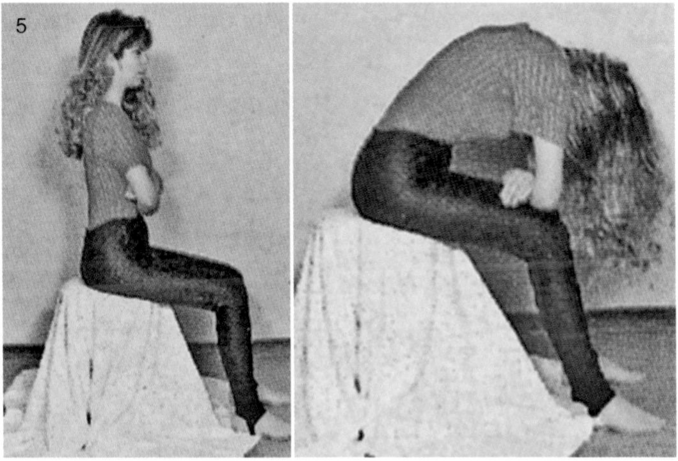

5. Sit down with your arms around the waist. Bend forward until your elbows touch the knees. Count up to five and rest. Repeat.

FIGURE 1.20 (continued)

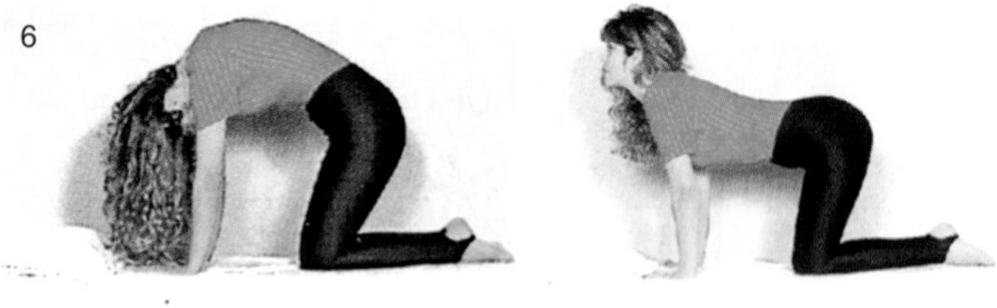

6. Place yourself as in picture 6. Bend your low back upwards and hold. Now bend it down and hold. Repeat.

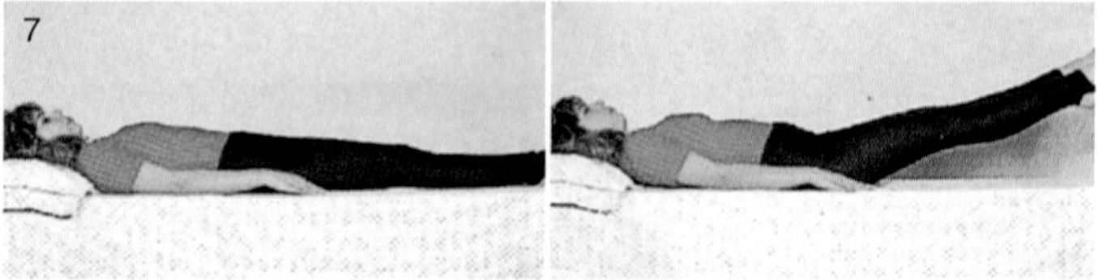

7. Strengthening your abdominal muscles. Lie on your back with your arms alongside you. Keep your knees straight and rise your heels about 20cm above the floor. Count up to five. Rest, relax and repeat.

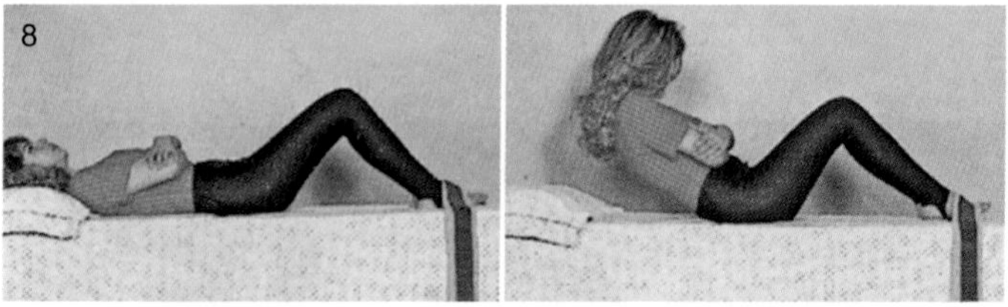

8. Strengthening your abdominal muscles. Lie on your back and strap your feet. Keep your knees bent to about 40 to 50°. Cross your arms in front of you and rise slowly from the bed as far as possible. Count up to five and slowly return to the initial position. Repeat.

FIGURE 1.20 (continued)

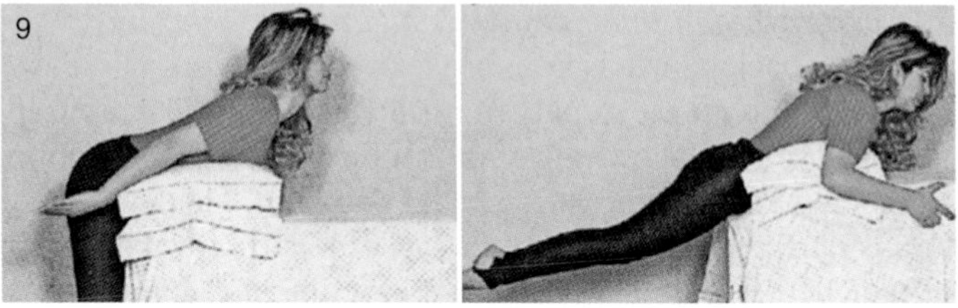

9. Bend over a table, with a pillow under your tummy. Hold to the table and rise your legs from the floor. Count up to three and rest. Rise your body from the table. Rest. Repeat.

Other means of protecting your back

1. Body weight. Excess body weight demands too much effort from your back, wearing out your bones and tiring your muscles. It is essential that you keep an appropriate body weight. (As an approximate rule, your weight in Kg should not exceed the number of cm of your height, above 1 m. Example: height 156cm. Ideal maximum weight ~56Kg)

2. Mattress and pillow. Be aware of soft mattresses! They may seem comfortable but they will not keep your back in a healthy position. Avoid sleeping on your stomach. Your will appreciate it.

3. Seating. Try to seat up straight, hold your back against the seat and get it close to the table. Use a lumbar support if needed. Always try to seat facing your working area, especially for prolonged tasks.

4. Bending down. Whenever possible, try to bend your knees and keep your back straight.

5. Standing. When required to stand up for long periods, use a a support to keep one of your feet about 15cm above the floor level. This will help your back to rest.

6. Footware. Give preference to shoes with about 2 cm of heel height.

7. Carrying weights. To shift and carry weights, use rule nº 4. Carry the weight close to your body. Whenever possible distribute the weight equally between your arms.

8. Rest. Try to distribute your workload during the day and plan periods of rest. Lie on your back and stretch out. A pillow under your knees may help your back to relax.

Perform these exercises regularly.
Help yourself!

FIGURE 1.20 (continued)

3. Analgesics, anti-inflammatories and muscle relaxants

In low back pain, a vicious circle of pain and muscle spasm often sets in: intense, repeated nociceptive stimuli caused by the disease result in exaggerated reflex muscle contraction, which accentuates and perpetuates the pain. This phenomenon is particularly important in cases of acute low back pain in which the muscle spasm may be clinically apparent. In these circumstances, it is important to relieve the pain as much as possible, not only for the patient's comfort but also for the physiopathological resolution of the clinical condition. We should opt for ordinary analgesics and save anti-inflammatories for more resistant cases. Muscle relaxants are particularly useful for exaggerated reflex muscle contraction.

Treatment of Ordinary Mechanical Low Back Pain

General Guidelines

Royal College of General Practitioners, UK[8]

Assessment

- Carry out diagnostic triage.
- X-rays are not routinely indicated in simple backache.
- Consider the psychological factors.

Medication

- Prescribe analgesics at regular intervals and not p.r.n.
- Start with paracetamol. If inadequate, replace with NSAIDs.
- Finally consider adding a short course of muscle relaxant.
- Avoid strong opioids if possible.
- Bed rest.
- Do not recommend or use bed rest as a treatment in simple low back pain.

[8]For more information or to access the latest version: http://rcgp.org.uk

- Some patients may be confined to bed for a few days as a consequence of their pain, but this should not be considered a treatment.

Advice on staying active

- Advise patients to stay as active as possible and to continue normal daily activities.
- Advise patients to increase their physical activities progressively over a few days or weeks.
- If a patient is working, then advice to stay at work or return to work as soon as possible is probably beneficial.

Manipulation

- Consider manipulative treatment in the first six weeks of an acute episode for patients who need additional help with pain relief or who are failing to return to normal activities.

Physical therapy

- Referral for physiotherapy/rehabilitation should be considered for patients who have not returned to ordinary activities and work by 6 weeks.

Psychological aspects

- Psychological, social and economic factors play an important role in chronic low back pain and physical disability. They influence the patient's response to treatment and rehabilitation.
- Psychological factors are important much earlier than we first thought.

In persistent, chronic cases, small doses of antidepressants (e.g. amitriptyline) may be very helpful in pain control.

4. Physical therapy

The local application of wet heat has a very useful relaxing effect, especially in acute low back pain. In the same way, a gentle local massage can help to relieve muscle contracture. Patients and their families can do this themselves at home with very little instruction (in a hot bath for example). Physical therapy may be necessary in cases that are particularly severe or resistant to simple measures. Manipulation of the spine by an experienced therapist may be very useful in the initial stages (<4 weeks) of an acute episode.

Physiotherapy sessions can be useful in dealing with chronic low back pain with incapacitating flare-ups, but the patient must also be committed to exercises regularly. Visits to physical therapy centers should always be used to educate the patient and not only for passive treatment sessions.

When Should the Patient be Referred to a Specialist?

(Most patients with low back pain can and should be treated by their GP.) All inflammatory back pain of unexplained causes.

Whenever there is reason to suspect an underlying systemic cause.

When there is neurological deficit that persists after conservative treatment.

In acute mechanical back pain if intense pain persists after 4-6 weeks of conservative treatment.

In chronic mechanical low back pain, if incapacitating pain persists in spite of an integrated plan of general care.

Chapter 2
Regional Syndromes
The Hip

The hip joint and the adjacent muscles and ligaments are often the site of disease. Given the importance of these structures in walking, their involvement can be an important cause of disability and suffering. Regional conditions can also seriously impair sexual activity. Given its deep location, physical examination of the hip is more about examining the joint movements than palpation but history and examination remain the pillar of most common diagnoses involving the hip.

Functional Anatomy

The hip joint consists of the femoral head and the acetabulum of the iliac bone (or hip bone). The depth of the acetabulum is increased by the acetabular labrum, a ring-shaped fibrocartilaginous structure that forms a tight collar around the femoral head. The labrum has a space in its lower part through which the transverse ligament passes, taking blood vessels to the inside of the joint.

The joint is covered by a resistant capsule that inserts around the acetabulum and the lateral end of the femoral neck, which is thus located inside the joint. The capsule is reinforced anteriorly, inferiorly and posteriorly by strong ligaments. Stability is increased by the muscles and ligamentum teres, an intra-articular ligament which arises from the acetabular rim and inserts into the vertex of the femoral head.

J.A.P. da Silva, A.D. Woolf, *Rheumatology of the Lower Limbs in Clinical Practice*, DOI 10.1007/978-1-4471-2253-1_2,

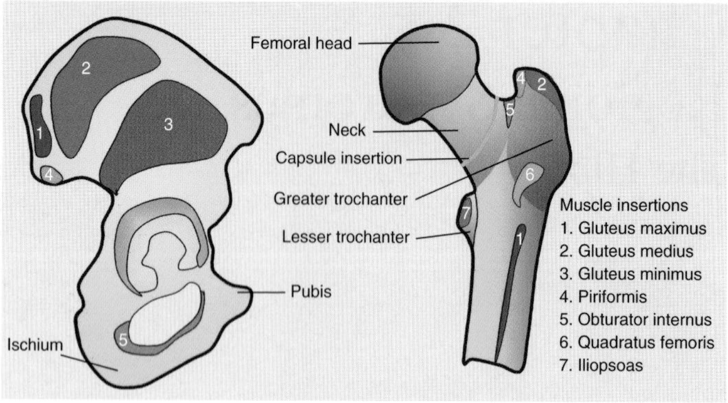

FIGURE 2.1 Muscle insertions on the iliac bone and proximal femur (Simplified scheme posterior aspect, right side)

The joint is deep-set and surrounded by powerful muscles that join the iliac bone and the proximal femur. Figure 2.1 shows the local muscle insertions. Several muscles insert into the superior, posterior and internal face of the trochanter. These muscles are responsible for abduction and external rotation of the thigh (piriform, internal obturator, superior and inferior gemelli, and quadriceps femoris). The external aspect of the greater trochanter is covered by the trochanteric bursa with extensions between the insertion fibers of the external rotators at the posterior and superior edge of the trochanter (Fig. 2.2). This area is often the site of painful inflammation. Given that it is not easy to distinguish bursitis from tendonitis on clinical grounds, we will use the expression "burso-tendonitis."

The sciatic nerve, which originates in the roots of L4 to S3, leaves the pelvis through the great sciatic foramen formed between the iliac bone and the sacrum, passing under the piriform muscle, which can produce pseudo-sciatic pain when inflamed.

The ischiotibial muscles (semimembranous, semitendinous and femoral biceps) insert into the ischium. The first two join the

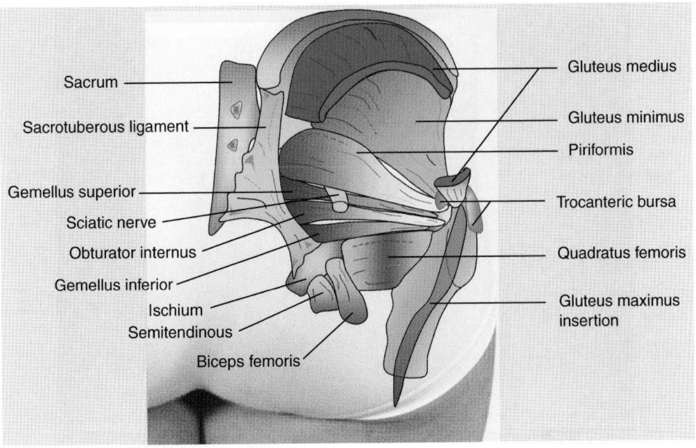

FIGURE 2.2 Muscles inserted posteriorly to the great trochanter and trochanteric bursa

iliac to the anterointernal face of the tibia. The biceps inserts into the lateral condyle of the tibia and head of the fibula. The ischium is covered by a bursa that can become inflamed causing local pain when sitting.

The iliotibial fascia, which is the direct continuation of the tensor fascia lata, extends along the lateral face of the thigh from the iliac crest to the external tubercle of the tibia. Powerful muscles insert into it and can cause excessive tension and pain.

The joint is capable of flexion (120°, diminishing with age), extension (about 30°), external rotation (60°), internal rotation (30°–40°), abduction (about 45°) and adduction (about 30°).

Flexion depends mainly on the iliopsoas muscle, which is innervated by L2/3. Extension is mainly the task of the gluteus maximus and the ischiotibials, which depend on L4/5 and S1/2, respectively. External rotation is induced by the gluteus maximus, piriform and quadriceps femoris (L4/5 and S1). Internal rotation is mainly the responsibility of the gluteus minimus (L4/5 and S1). Figure 1.2 shows the dermatomes of the hip.

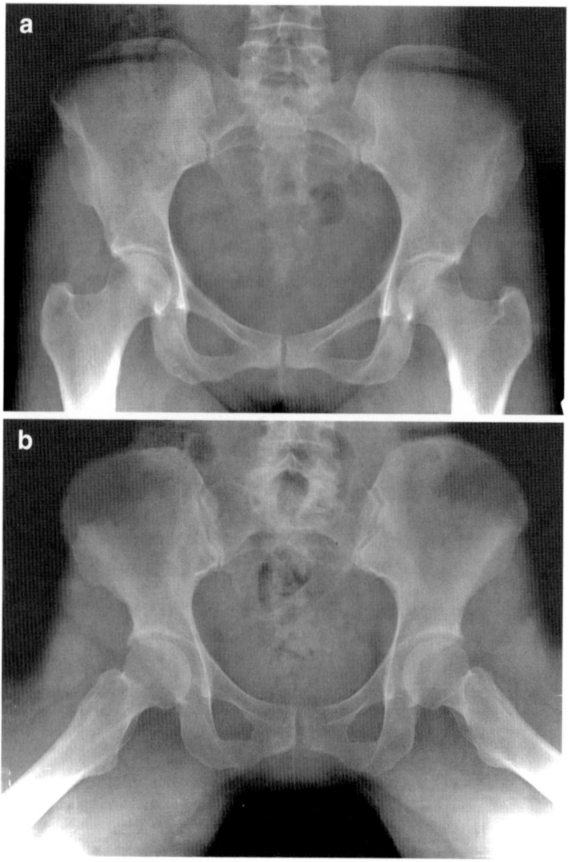

FIGURE 2.3 Radiological anatomy of the pelvis. (**a**) Antero-posterior view – the hip and sacro-iliac joints. Search for lytic or sclerotic focal lesions, as well as fractures, in the iliac bones and proxi mal part of the femurs. (**b**) Frog-leg view. Additional evaluation of the hip joints and of the femoral head. Some fractures of the proximal femur will only be detected with this view

Radiological Anatomy

From an anteroposterior view (Fig. 2.3a) we can see the hip joints: size and regularity of the articular space and surfaces, morphology of the femoral head, and coverage of the head by

TABLE 2.1 Common causes of hip pain

Etiology	Clinical clues
Referred pain	Pain radiating from the lumbar spine, sacroiliac joints, appendix and urinary tract Poorly defined Associated manifestations Normal local examination
Trochanteric burso-tendonitis	Pain in the lateral aspect of the hip Worse at night (lying on ipsilateral side) Frequent pseudo-sciatic radiation Typical pain on local pressure
Osteoarthritis	Mechanical pain Progressive onset Limited active and passive mobility Predominates in the elderly
Arthritis	Rarely monoarthritis Inflammatory pain Suggestive general context Limited active and passive mobility
Tendonitis of the adductors	Pain in the inguinal region Exacerbated by forced abduction Often accompanies hip disease Typical pain on local pressure Specific provocation maneuvers

the acetabulum. This is also the best routine angle for evaluating the sacroiliac joints. Look at their lower third and assess the size of the space and the definition, density and regularity of the articular surfaces. Look for focal alterations in the bone density of the iliacs and proximal femur (lytic or sclerotic lesions).

The lateral radiograph (Fig. 2.3b) shows changes in the joint space and the morphology of the head or even fractures that may not be evident when viewed anteroposteriorly.

Common Causes of Pain in the Hip Area

Referred pain, burso-tendonitis and osteoarthritis are the most common causes of isolated hip area pain (Table 2.1). The joint is often involved in polyarticular disease, in which case the clinical context suggests the diagnosis and suitable investigation.

A thorough local examination is always essential, not only to clarify the nature of the local involvement, but also to assess the indication for local therapy adjuvant to the systemic treatment.

The Enquiry

The Exact Location of the Pain

The location of the pain is an important clue for diagnosis. Hip joint pain is usually located deep in the groin along the inguinal ligament, although in some patients it is felt deep in the buttocks.

Pain referred from the spine and sacroiliac joints, which is probably the most common in clinical practice, affects the buttocks diffusely. Occasionally pain of this origin is accompanied by dysesthesia.

Trochanteric burso-tendonitis may be extremely misleading. Usually, the patient (typically an obese, middle-aged woman), locates the pain in the lateral aspect of the hip. In some cases, however, the pain radiates to the buttocks and even down to the knee, along the external aspect of the thigh. In tendonitis of the adductors, the pain is confined to the medial aspect of the inguinal region.

The Rhythm of the Pain

Pain due to osteoarthritis and synovitis has the expected mechanical and inflammatory rhythms, respectively. The rhythm of referred pain depends on the cause. In most cases it is mechanical, and is often associated with chronic mechanical backache. The pain from sacroiliitis, however, often involves the buttocks, with a typically inflammatory rhythm.

Pain caused by lesions of the soft tissues is more variable in rhythm and is mostly associated with walking and postures that cause tension or compression of the inflamed structures.

Exacerbating Factors

Exacerbation of pain when the patient is lying on their side in bed is strongly suggestive of ipsilateral trochanteric burso-tendonitis. The pain from tendonitis of the adductors worsens with abduction, when getting into a car for example. Both may be exacerbated by walking, but not by flexion of the spine.

On the contrary, this last symptom suggests pain radiating from the lumbar spine. Exacerbation of the pain by Valsava's maneuvers also suggests a lumbar cause. Note, however, that more anxious patients may describe this feature in other situations.

Form of Onset and Clinical Context

The onset of osteoarthritis is usually very slow and progressive. As a rule, the patient goes to the doctor only after several years of recurrent episodes of pain of growing intensity. Most patients with hip osteoarthritis have the same disease in other load-bearing joints, particularly the knees. It usually affects the elderly.

Monoarthritis of the hip is very rare. In most cases, hip synovitis appears in the context of an oligo- or polyarticular inflammatory disease and can be found in practically all types of arthritis. Monoarthritis of the hip should be considered septic until proven otherwise. In either case, the onset is relatively quick (days or weeks).

Radiating pain is usually accompanied by chronic or recurrent acute low back pain, which should be taken into account, even if the patient focuses his or her description on the hip area. Occasionally, a patient with hip region pain and fever may have appendicitis or a urinary infection.

Trochanteric burso-tendonitis is extremely common in clinical practice and often appears with no associated pathology. It may simulate sciatica. Remember to exclude this possibility whenever you are thinking of sciatic pain!

Conversely, tendonitis of the adductors most often accompanies a recent exacerbation of hip joint disease. Even in these situations, it often dominates the patient's clinical condition, making its identification and treatment very rewarding, even if the joint disease persists.

Hip region pain is also common in patients with fibromyalgia. Four of the typically sensitive points of fibromyalgia are located around this area. Pay attention to the context of generalized pain.

The Regional Examination

Inspection

Inspection is not very productive in diseases of the hip, as it is a deep joint protected by muscle. Periarticular lesions are not usually accompanied by visible swelling or redness. Clinical assessment of the hip joint is based essentially on mobilization.

Leg length discrepancy, described in the previous chapter, may also cause hip pain and should be considered.

Mobilization

Mobilization of the hip as described in the general rheumatologic examination is sufficient for exploring this joint. Mobilization is passive while the patient is lying on their back relaxed.

1. We first induce passive elevation of the leg, thus testing the sciatic nerve, then assess flexion, extension, internal and external rotation, abduction and adduction.

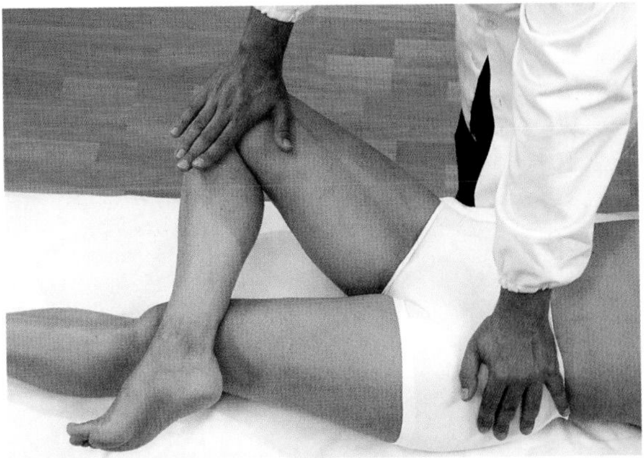

FIGURE 2.4 Forced abduction with external rotation. Pain in the insertion of the adductor muscles close the pubic symphysis suggest adductor tendonitis

Note that angles given as normal for these movements vary from one person to another, and tend to diminish with age. Always make a comparison with the other side.

Hip osteoarthritis starts with painful limitation of internal rotation and abduction, and affects the other movements later. Do not forget that extension is assessed while forcing flexion of the contralateral hip (Thomas's test).

In hip joint synovitis, all movements are painful.

In referred pain, mobilization of the hip, especially forced flexion, may cause pain in the lumbar region, possibly radiating to the buttocks.

Patients with trochanteric bursitis-tendonitis often complain of pain on forced internal rotation, though it is not always present.

In tendonitis of the adductors, the pain is more intense during forced abduction. Where appropriate, this condition should be explored with more specific maneuvers:

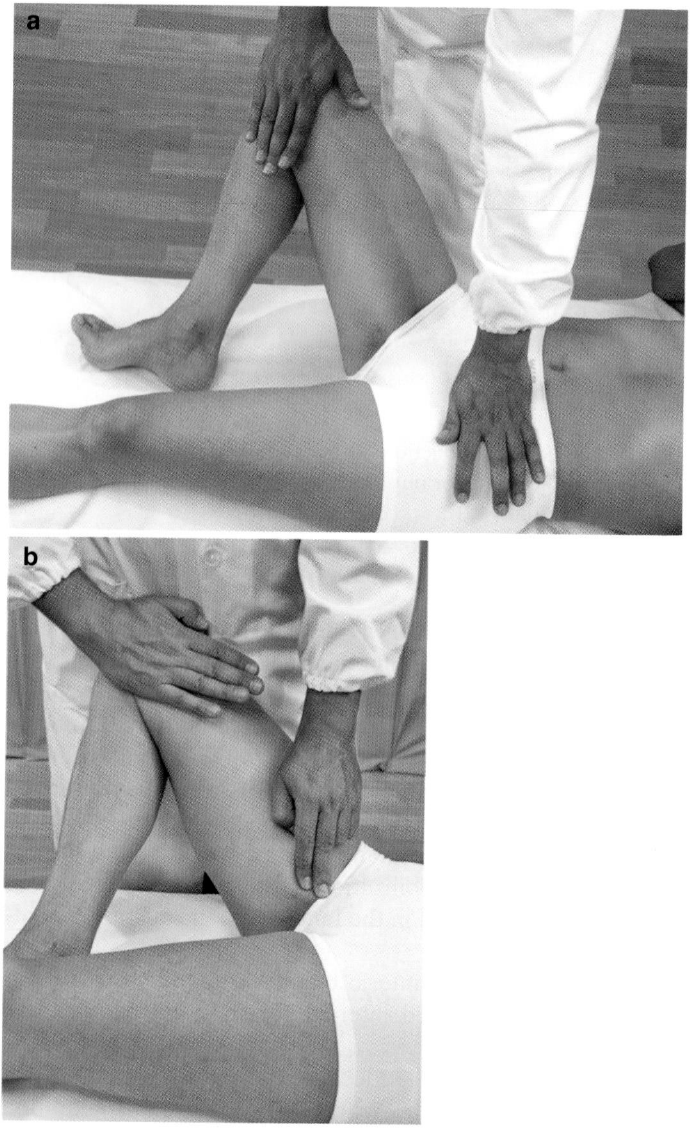

FIGURE 2.5 (**a**) Resisted adduction of the thigh. Pain the inguinal area suggests adductor tendonitis. (**b**) Tenderness at the tendon insertion also supports the diagnosis

2. The patient crosses his legs, placing his foot on the outside of the contralateral knee. The observer then forces abduction (Fig. 2.4). This maneuver causes pain on the inside of the inguinal region, in the presence of tendonitis of the adductors.

3. With his knee flexed to about 90° and his foot on the examining table, the patient is asked to adduct his knee, against the observer's resistance (Fig. 2.5). Pain in the inguinal region suggests

Palpation

The hip joint is not directly palpable, and so we cannot directly assess the existence of swelling, effusion, heat or even crepitus.

Palpation is used mainly to examine the points of common periarticular involvement:

4. Bursa and trochanter muscle insertions. Slide your fingers over the external aspect of the hip from the iliac crest, palpating deeply. Note the bony promontory formed by the greater trochanter. Exert firm pressure on the external face of this promontory. This is where the trochanteric bursa is located. Also palpate along the superior and posterior edges of the trochanter. This is the most common location of pain, suggesting inflammation of the muscle insertions of the abductors (Fig. 2.6). Quite often this area of tenderness extends distally well into the fascia lata.

   If in doubt as to the intensity of the pain and palpation, examine the other side.

Note that there may be pain on palpation in the absence of local inflammation. It is a frequent finding in fibromyalgia.

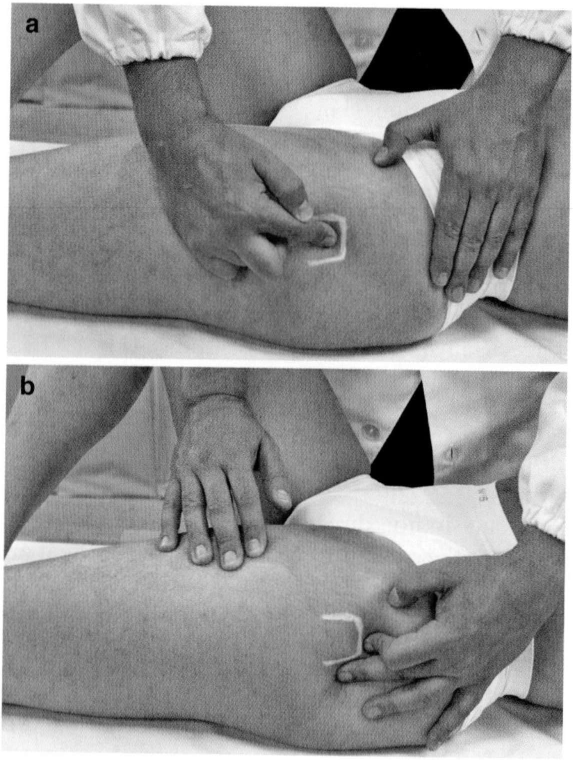

FIGURE 2.6 Palpating the trochanteric bursa (**a**) and muscle insertions in the vicinity (**b**)

Clinical assessment of the hip is not complete without an examination of the lumbar spine and the knee. A careful abdominal and pelvic examination is also indicated on occasions.

FIGURE 2.7 Radiograph of the right hip – Clinical case "Mechanical hip pain (I)". Note the complete loss of joint space associated with subchondral sclerosis, focal radiolucent areas (geodes or subchondral cysts). These are typical features of osteoarthritis

Typical Cases

2.A. Mechanical Hip Pain (I)

Alfredo Porfírio, an 82-year old farmer, had been monitored by his doctor for years with polyarticular osteoarthritis involving the spine, hips and knees, which was being treated with analgesics and anti-inflammatories. The pain was typical: exacerbated by exercise and walking and relieved by rest, with no significant morning stiffness. He had been offered replacement surgery for his right hip, but he had declined because of the many associated diseases that he had as well as the advice of his cardiologist. He came to us because the pain in his right hip had recently worsened, further limiting his walking and also making it difficult to drive. He also said that the pain persisted at night in the right inguinal region.

He walked with small steps and rotation of the pelvis. An examination of his hips showed extreme limitation of mobility in abduction, adduction, internal and external rotation and extension. He could manage about 90 flexion. There were no doubts about the diagnosis from the pelvic x-ray that he had with him (Fig. 2.7).

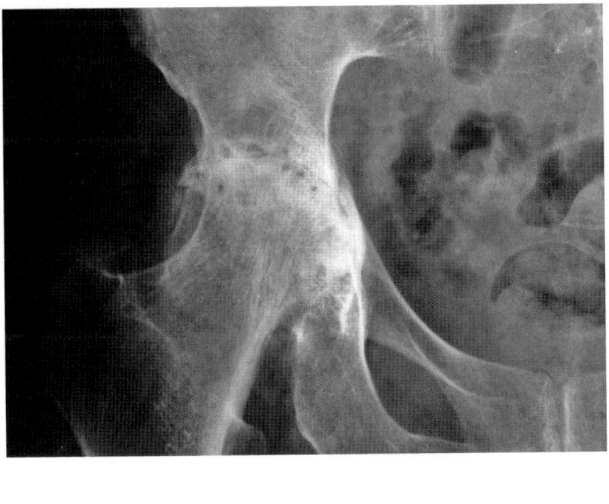

Was the situation completely clear?
What could have caused the recent deterioration?

Abduction triggered intense pain in the anterior aspect of the right hip and particularly in the internal part of the inguinal region. Resisted adduction was very painful. Palpation identified intense pain at the superior insertion of the adductors of the right thigh. Most of his pain could be caused by tendonitis of the adductors, a common complication of hip osteoarthritis.

What treatment would you suggest?
We carefully administered a local injection of methylprednisolone and xylocaine around the tendon. He noticed the difference almost immediately with a significant reduction in pain on passive mobilization and when walking. This relief, which enabled him to go back to his normal daily activities, lasted for about a year, after which we repeated the procedure. For economic and personal reasons, Mr. Porfírio had not taken the physical therapy that we had recommended.

Osteoarthritis of the Hip
Main Points
This condition is common in men and women over 50, though it can appear earlier.

Predisposing factors include childhood hip disease (Legg-Perthes disease, slipped femoral epiphysis, and congenital hip dysplasia), acetabular dysplasia and hard physical labor (farmers, miners).

It causes mechanical pain in the inguinal region, which can radiate to the knee or buttocks. Brief stiffness after rest is common. It is often accompanied by osteoarthritis of other weightbearing joints.

Clinical examination reveals pain and limited mobility, especially of internal rotation. Secondary shortening of the affected leg may occur.

Progression varies: most patients will worsen slowly with growing limitations to mobility.

X-rays show typical signs of osteoarthritis: polar loss of articular space, subchondral sclerosis (sometimes with subchondral geodes and cysts), and osteophytes.

Treatment is conservative in the initial stages:

- Analgesics or anti-inflammatories
- Well cushioned footwear to absorb the shock of walking
- A walking stick or crutch on the opposite arm
- Encouraging physical exercise and self-sufficiency
- Physical therapy in more advanced cases

Although there are no solid criteria as to the best time for a total hip replacement, we consider that it is indicated if the patient cannot sleep, walk or work because of the osteoarthritis despite suitable analgesia. The results are usually highly satisfactory.

Tendonitis of the Hip Adductors

Main Points

It appears most commonly in patients with hip osteoarthritis, but can occur on its own in athletes, for example.

It causes pain in the internal part of the inguinal region, aggravated by abduction of the hip.

The diagnosis can be made if there is pain over the tendon on palpation, forced abduction and resisted adduction.

Inguinal pain may be caused by a hernia.

Treatment is conservative, aiming at strengthening the muscles and local rest. It is important to relieve the local and hip pain to facilitate muscle relaxation.

In more intense or stubborn cases, a careful local injection can be administered.

Typical Cases

2.B. Mechanical Hip Pain (II)

Leonor Rodrigues, a retired teacher aged 58, came to us with pain in her right hip, that had been getting progressively worse over the last three years. It hurt when she walked, getting progressively worse with continued use and preventing her from taking the evening walks she enjoyed so much. The pain was relieved by rest. It was diffuse and imprecisely located in the groin and the buttocks, sometimes radiating to the posterior aspect of the thigh. She also complained of an old, fluctuating mechanical backache, which "she was used to." Occasionally, she had pain in her knees when walking upstairs but it was bearable. She took anti-inflammatories when the pain was more intense, with moderate relief.

The systematic enquiry revealed no relevant findings.

The general examination showed an obese, good-humored woman (weight 72 Kg, height 1.50 m), with slow, difficult movements of the lower limbs. Forced flexion of the lumbar spine caused pain. Extension was also painful, radiating vaguely to the buttocks. Her arms were normal. Mobility of the hip joints was notably preserved. Forced flexion caused lumbar pain and reproduced the spontaneous complaints. An examination of her knees revealed crepitus in the patellofemoral compartment. Palpation around the hip did not reveal any painful areas. The summary neurological examination was normal.

How would you explain this patient's hip pain?
Were any diagnostic tests necessary?

This information led us to consider that it was probably radiated pain from the chronic mechanical back pain, most likely associated with spondyloarthrosis and osteoarthritis of the facet joints. We gave the patient appropriate advice, stressing the need for regular exercise and care with her posture because of her spine. We carefully explained the need to lose weight, emphasizing the relationship between obesity and osteoarthritis of the spine and knee. We suggested she take simple analgesics as required to relieve the pain and enable her to exercise. We recommended that she join an exercise or stretching class.

Referred Hip Pain

Main Points

Hip pain can radiate from the lumbar spine, sacroiliac joints and abdominal organs (pelvis, urether, bladder, appendicitis or diverticulitis in contact with the iliopsoas muscle[1]).

Its location is diffuse and ill defined, predominating in the buttocks when it comes from the spine and in abdomen and groin if caused by intra-abdominal pathology.

Degenerative pathologies of the spine and hip often coexist, but they can occur separately, requiring different treatment.

When dealing with hip pain, always explore the lumbar spine and sacroiliac joints, along with the abdomen and pelvis.

A detailed local physical examination fails to explain the pain.

A general rheumatologic and abdominal examination is the key to the diagnosis.

Treatment is aimed at the underlying condition.

Typical Cases

2.C. Nocturnal Hip Pain (I)

According to the patient, a 52-year old personal assistant, the worst thing about her pain was that it stopped her from sleeping. She was able to rest on her back, but could

[1]Note that in these last cases the patient may mention painful limitation of mobility of the hip and the pain may worsen with active and passive mobilization of the hip due to inflammation of the iliopsoas…

not bear the pain if she lay on her side. As this was her natural position, she would wake up several times during the night. The pain was bearable during the day. She had trouble getting up after sitting for a long time, but the pain soon went. She also had to be careful when sitting on the toilet, to avoid the pain, but the strain of defecation did not make it worse. She located the pain on the lateral face of both hip areas and denied any radiation.

She was generally healthy and was not taking any medication. Her doctor suspected that the cause was lumbar. However, a spinal x-ray did not show any significant anomalies, apart from a discreet degree of osteoarthritis.

Our examination of her spine revealed no alterations, although forced flexion caused slight pain in the posterior aspect of the thighs and knees.

Passive mobilization of the hips required great efforts to relax the patient, who was afraid that it would hurt. Having managed this, however, there was only slight pain in the posterolateral face of both hip areas during forced internal rotation. There was no limited mobility in any direction. Sciatic nerve stretch tests were negative.

Trochanteric Burso-Tendonitis

Main Points

This is an inflammatory process that affects the trochanteric bursa and/or the muscle insertions in the greater trochanter of the femur.

It is one of the most common causes of hip pain, predominating in middle-aged and elderly women.

The pain is felt in the external face of the hip and may radiate to the buttock and external face of the thigh.

It is exacerbated by lying on the ipsilateral side and walking.

It does not affect passive mobility of the hip, though it can cause some pain in extreme rotation. Firm local palpation reproduces the symptoms.

Obesity, leg length discrepancy, hip joint disease and demanding exercise like running predispose to this pathology.

No diagnostic tests are necessary (ultrasound scans often give false positives and negatives).

Treatment is conservative: local rest, relaxation, topical anti-inflammatories and heat. SEE ABOVE

Physical therapy or local injection may be necessary in cases with more intense symptoms or that are resistant to basic treatment.

What could be happening?

Would you look for any additional information from the physical examination?

Palpation of the trochanteric region triggered intense pain, limited to the external face of the trochanter on the left side but much more extensive on the right (superior and posterior border of the trochanter and an adjacent area of the fascia lata).

The general examination and the examination of the other joints were normal.

What is your diagnosis?

How would you proceed?

We decided that it was bilateral trochanteric burso-tendonitis, more extensive on the right side. We explained the condition to the patient and reassured her. We prescribed a topical anti-inflammatory for her to apply three times a day after local heat. We referred her to a physiotherapy centre for muscle relaxation exercises. After the third week, the patient was much better and said that the pain on the left side had cleared up though there was still some discomfort on the right. An examination of this area revealed pain on pressure, now limited to the superior edge of the trochanter. We administered a local injection of anaesthetic and corticosteroid, which relieved the symptoms.

Typical Cases

2.D. Nocturnal Hip Pain (II)

Pain in his left hip finally forced António, a 42-year old, self-employed carpenter, to take time off to go to the doctor.

The pain had begun about three months before and had deteriorated rapidly. It was located all around his hip region, predominating in the lateral and anterior face. It was particularly severe when he got up after rest and improved slowly with movement. It persisted at night, though it was less intense. It was accompanied by morning stiffness for about 40 minutes. Anti-inflammatories, which he had been taking for several years "for his back," did not help very much.

Could the backache be related to the hip pain? How could we investigate this?

Our enquiry into the back pain was interesting. It also had an inflammatory rhythm, similar to the hip pain. It had started three years before and responded well to the anti-inflammatory that he took at night.

He denied any complaints in other joints. Our systematic enquiry was negative, including questions about any skin, mucosal or intestinal changes. The rest of his personal history was not relevant. His father had suffered from psoriasis, however.

We found no anomalies on general examination, including signs of psoriasis. Mobility of the lumbar spine was frankly reduced, with a Schober of 10–13.2 cm. Palpation and mobilization of the sacroiliac joints triggered pain on the right.

The left hip joint was painful on active and passive mobilization in all directions. Passive mobility was limited by pain.

What possibilities does this clinical condition suggest?
What additional studies would you request?

The pain was typically inflammatory and accompanied by painful limitation of mobility, strongly suggesting arthritis. The back pain, which might seem quite normal in a physical worker, was also inflammatory – an alarm signal. The patient had no systemic manifestations, but his father's history of psoriasis was important. The possibility of psoriatic arthritis, with predominant axial involvement and affecting the hip had to be explored.

We requested plain films of the lumbar and thoracic spine (2 views), an anteroposterior view of the pelvis and lateral views of both hips. We also asked for routine blood tests, including acute phase reactants, full blood count and liver tests in preparation for disease-modifying treatment. We also ordered a technetium bone scan because of the difficulty involved in the physical examination of these deep joints.

His sedimentation rate was elevated at 47 mm in the first hour. The full blood count, liver enzymes and routine tests were normal. The spinal x-ray showed no alterations. His hips were also radiologically normal (which did not exclude synovitis, in view of the short time since onset). Figure 2.8 shows the x-ray of the pelvis. The bone scan performed three months later showed increased uptake in the right sacroiliac joint.

In view of these results, we decided that our tentative diagnosis had been confirmed. Given that the involvement

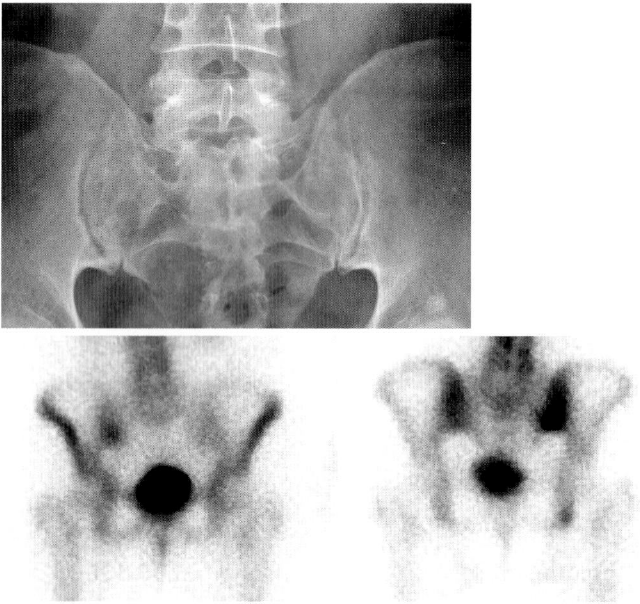

FIGURE 2.8 X-Ray of the pelvis – Clinical case "Nocturnal hip pain (II)." Note the blurring of the right sacroiliac joint margin, with subchondral sclerosis and erosions. This demonstrates the presence of asymmetrical sacro-iliítis, quite compatible with psoriatic arthritis. Bone scintigraphy reveals increased uptake of the radiotracer around the right sacro-iliac joint. AV – Anterior view. PV – posterior view

was predominantly axial and, therefore would not be very responsive to disease-modifying drugs, we decided to continue treatment with anti-inflammatories and administer a local injection in the hip guided by ultrasound. We stressed the need for the patient to do regular exercises of the spine and to be aware of potential side effects of the medication.

The result was excellent, but we continued to monitor the patient, as the involvement of new joints might justify a different treatment.

Arthritis of the Hip
Main Points
Synovitis of the hip is suggested by:
- Local inflammatory pain;
- Painful limitation of active and passive mobility;
- Elevated acute phase reactants;
- Circumferential loss of radiological articular space, with no subchondral sclerosis (appears later);
- Increased uptake of radiolabel on bone scintigraphy.

It normally appears in the context of more disseminated arthritis. When isolated, it should be considered septic until proven otherwise: a rheumatologic emergency.

It requires differential diagnosis with osteoarthritis, periarticular lesions, sacroiliitis, avascular necrosis of the femoral head, …

Treatment depends on the underlying disease. Septic arthritis requires bacteriological diagnosis and urgent, sometimes surgical, treatment.

Persistent arthritis of the hip may justify an imaging-guided corticosteroid injection as a rapid way of reducing the inflammation and preventing irreversible sequelae.

Special Situations

Avascular (Previously called Aseptic) Necrosis of the Femoral Head

This is a relatively uncommon condition in clinical practice but requires timely diagnosis. It involves the loss of viability of a part of the femoral head bone and overlying cartilage due to ischemia. The ischemia alone causes pain that is sometimes incapacitating. The dead tissue collapses, causing irregularity on the articular surface, with or without the release of free intraarticular bodies, which will lead to the relentless development of osteoarthritis (Fig. 2.9).

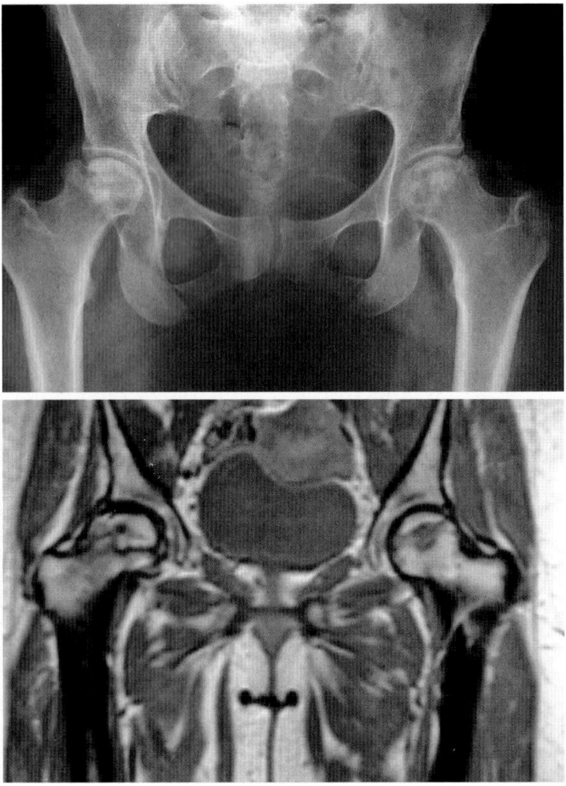

FIGURE 2.9 Bilateral aseptic necrosis of the femoral head. Note the deformity and sclerotic aspect of the femoral head. This patient, with systemic lupus, required bilateral hip replacement a few years later

It appears most frequently in young people with predisposing factors: chronic glucocorticoid treatment, systemic lupus erythematosus, antiphospholipid syndrome, alcoholism, diabetes mellitus, AIDS and local trauma. Sometimes no predisposing factors are identified.

Early diagnosis requires, above all, a high degree of suspicion. This condition is heralded by articular pain in the hip, with a variable rhythm, but often inflammatory. Mobility of the hip joint may be limited, even in the early stages of the disease. Radiographs should be from an anteroposterior projection

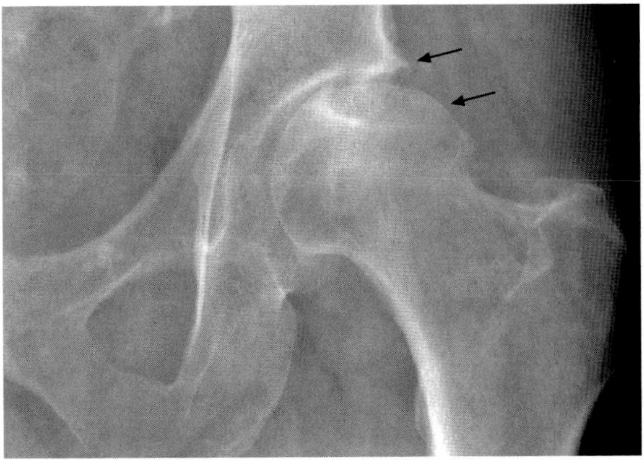

FIGURE 2.10 Aseptic necrosis of the left femoral head. Notice the focal sclerosis of the superior part of the femoral head with slight deformation and loss of continuity of the cortical layer. There are already features of secondary osteoarthritis: loss of joint space, subchondral sclerosis and early osteophytes (*arrows*)

and lateral, trying to identify subtle loss of the spherical shape of the femoral head (Fig. 2.10). This deformation becomes more marked over time. Ideally, however, the diagnosis should be made before any radiological changes, using magnetic resonance imaging (the earliest and most specific technique) (Fig. 2.11) or technetium bone scan.

If the diagnosis is confirmed a careful search for likely causes should be initiated. Treatment is based on analgesics. Ultimately, hip replacement may be required.

Meralgia Paresthetica

This is caused by compression of the lateral femoral cutaneous nerve in the vicinity of the anterosuperior iliac spine or where it exits the deep fascia in the anterior face of the thigh. It causes pain and paresthesia in the anterolateral aspect of the thigh (Fig. 2.12), often aggravated by certain positions, such as crossed legs. Accentuated obesity or tight clothes can precipitate the symptoms. The neurological examination may

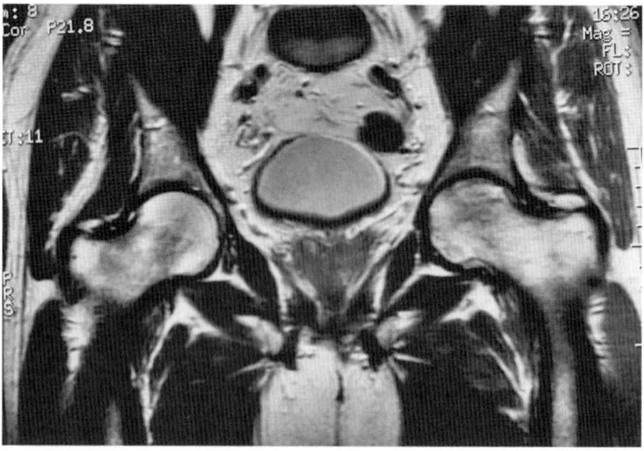

FIGURE 2.11 Aseptic necrosis of the femoral head – early phase. Magnetic resonance imaging shows a change of signal in the left femoral head – "crescent sign." The shape of the femoral head is still preserved and there are no signs of osteoarthritis

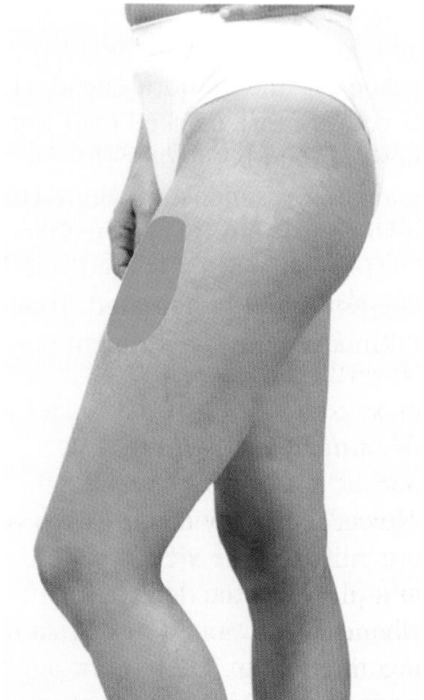

FIGURE 2.12 Area of hyposthesia or paraesthesia in meralgia paresthetica

reveal hypo- or hyperesthesia in the affected area. Palpation or percussion of the nerve's exit point just below the antero-superior iliac spine or at a point 10 cm below it can trigger pain. An electromyogram may confirm the diagnosis.

Treatment is aimed at removing the causes, if they have been identified. In their absence or if the symptoms persist, local injections or even surgical decompression may be necessary.

Iliopectineal Bursitis

The iliopectineal bursa is deep within the median part of the inguinal region between the anterior face of the articular capsule and the iliopsoas tendon. It communicates with the synovium of the hip joint in about 15% of people and can be involved in its inflammatory processes.

It causes pain in the anterior face of the thigh and inguinal region, which is aggravated by flexion of the thigh. Local palpation is painful. Plain films are normal. The diagnosis requires ultrasound or MRI scans.

Treatment is directed towards the associated hip disease, if any. Ultrasound-guided local injections may be very useful.

Fractures of the Proximal Femur and Pelvis

Many fractures of the proximal femur or pelvis are obvious, not only because of violent trauma required to sustain them but also because of the immediate functional disability that they cause. The radiographs usually leave no doubt. Nevertheless, fractures of the proximal femur are one of the most common types of osteoporotic fracture. In these cases, the trauma may be minimal or even non-existent. Many osteoporotic fractures occurring under the patient's weight get "stuck," i.e. the bone ends are compacted into each other. The disability is less marked and the fracture may not be detectable in a physical examination. We should consider this possibility whenever an elderly patient presents with acute pain in the inguinal region, especially if there are other risk factors for osteoporosis. Note that in an early x-ray, the fracture line may

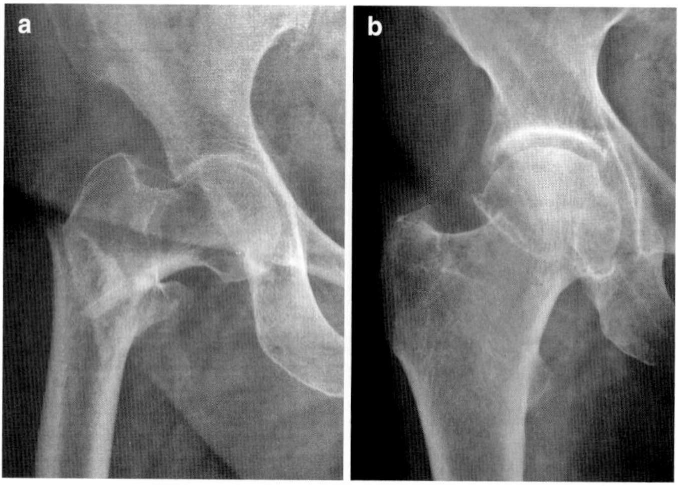

FIGURE 2.13 Osteoporotic fractures of the proximal femur. (**a**) In most cases, the fracture is obvious on the x-ray. (**b**) Bone endings may, however, be impacted making the diagnosis more difficult. Fractures may be obscurred by coexisting haematoma. (Courtesy: Prof. Fernando Fonseca)

be concealed by a local hematoma (Fig. 2.13), especially in compacted fractures.

Severe osteoporosis is also associated with factures of the iliac bone (namely in the iliopubic branch) and sacrum, which may occur spontaneously or after minimal trauma. These fractures cause deep, sometimes continuous disabling pain with no apparent cause. A careful x-ray examination in at least two planes and bone scanning may provide the key to the diagnosis.

Metastases and Paget's bone disease are other causes of pelvic pain to be considered in the elderly.

Diagnostic Tests

As always, clinical assessment takes first place and, in most cases, it is all we need to make a diagnosis and prescribe treatment.

Referred hip pain, trochanteric burso-tendonitis and tendonitis of the adductors all fall into this category. The x-rays will be normal in these conditions. Peritrochanteric calcification or irregular bone at the insertion of the adductors is occasionally visible. This reinforces the diagnosis, but does not change the treatment.

Imaging

An anteroposterior x-ray of the pelvis is usually sufficient for studying the hip and sacroiliac joints. Suspected aseptic necrosis, Legg-Perthes disease or slipped femoral epiphysis may justify lateral films so that we can evaluate the sphericity or dislocation of the epiphysis.

Radiographs in osteoarthritis show the same typical characteristics of this condition in any location (Fig. 2.14a): focal loss of joint space, subchondral sclerosis and osteophytes. In some cases, such as aseptic necrosis, the femoral head may appear atrophic, reduced in size, with no osteophytes.

In osteoarthritis, the loss of articular space predominates in the superior pole of the femoral head and the adjacent area of the acetabulum. Conversely, in inflammatory arthritides, the loss of articular space is diffuse, without subchondral sclerosis or osteophytes, unless there is secondary osteoarthritis (Fig. 2.14b). In advanced cases, synovitis may be accompanied by erosions of the periphery of the femoral head. Septic arthritis causes rapidly progressive destruction, with loss of bone definition.

MRI scans are only justified to investigate possible aseptic necrosis or even rarer conditions, in the sphere of specialized care.

Situations involving persistent, incapacitating pain that are still undefined after a basic clinical examination and tests may benefit from bone scanning, which can help clarify situations of arthritis, aseptic necrosis or rarer conditions like osteoid osteoma and algodystrophy (circumscribed osteoporosis of the hip – see Chap. 4).

Ultrasound scans are most indicated in the study of soft tissue lesions. However, clinical examination of the hip is quite specific while ultrasound is relatively unreliable in this area.

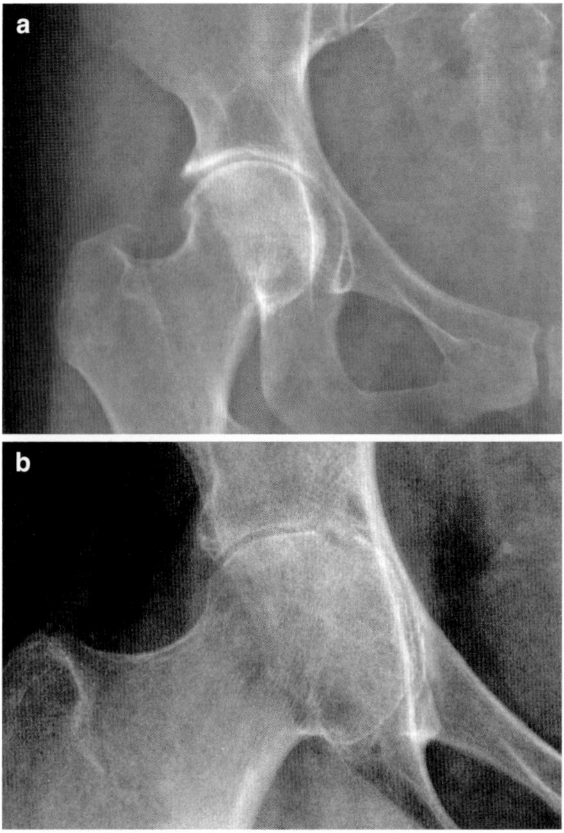

FIGURE 2.14 (**a**) Hip osteoarthritis. Note the loss of joint space, predominating in the upper pole, subchondral sclerosis and osteophytes. (**b**) Inflammatory arthritis of the hip: joint space loss is uniform and there is no subchondral sclerosis or osteophyte formation

Other Tests

Laboratory tests, such as the sedimentation rate, C reactive protein, rheumatoid factor, antiphospholipid antibodies, synovial biopsy and analysis of the synovial fluid may be indicated in cases of arthritis of unknown origin or aseptic necrosis, usually in a specialized context.

Treatment

The initial treatment of most causes of hip pain is within the reach of General Practitioners and has already been described.

The use of simple analgesics and, possibly, anti-inflammatories is often justified and worth while. Treatment of referred pain is determined by the cause. Treatment of hip osteoarthritis follows the general rules for this condition. A diagnosis or strong suspicion of arthritis of unknown origin justifies referring the patient to a specialist as soon as possible.

The patient should always be encouraged to take physical exercise compatible with his or her physical ability. Reinforcing lumbar and abdominal muscles and the quadriceps with simple exercises at home is excellent for relieving the pain and maintaining long-term function. Particularly debilitated patients and those with resistant tendonitis or bursitis may benefit from physical therapy.

When Should the Patient be Referred to a Specialist?

Whenever arthritis of unknown cause is suspected.

Reasonable suspicion of aseptic necrosis of the femoral head.

Whenever the pain is still incapacitating in spite of appropriate basic treatment.

Physical therapy can be very useful for patients with persistent periarticular lesions or moderate or severe osteoarthritis, when surgery is contraindicated.

In cases of osteoarthritis or avascular necrosis, total hip replacement should be considered, when the pain and loss of mobility cause substantial functional limitation, after excluding periarticular causes of aggravation.

Chapter 3
Regional Syndromes
The Knee

The knee is the largest and one of the most complex joints in the human body. With a large synovium and subject to extreme mechanical demands, it is highly prone to both mechanical and inflammatory lesions. Diseases of the knees, such as osteoarthritis, and lesions of the meniscus and ligaments, are some of the most common causes of disability.

Functional Anatomy

The knee joint brings together three bones: the distal end of the femur via the femoral condyles, the proximal end of the tibia, through the tibial plates (or condyles) and the patella, the largest sesamoid bone in the body. The menisci, which consist of crescent-shaped, triangular in section hyaline cartilages, partially separate the articular surfaces of the femur and tibia. They adhere to the interior face of the capsule and help the joint to glide and remain stable while absorbing a substantial part of the joint's mechanical load (Fig. 3.1). The menisci are subject to multiple trauma due to friction and "trapping," and are a common cause of symptoms.

We can think of the knee joint as having three compartments: medial tibiofemoral, lateral tibiofemoral and patellofemoral.

The articular capsule completely surrounds these joints, inserting in the borders of the patella and along the borders of

J.A.P. da Silva, A.D. Woolf, *Rheumatology of the Lower Limbs in Clinical Practice*, DOI 10.1007/978-1-4471-2253-1_3,

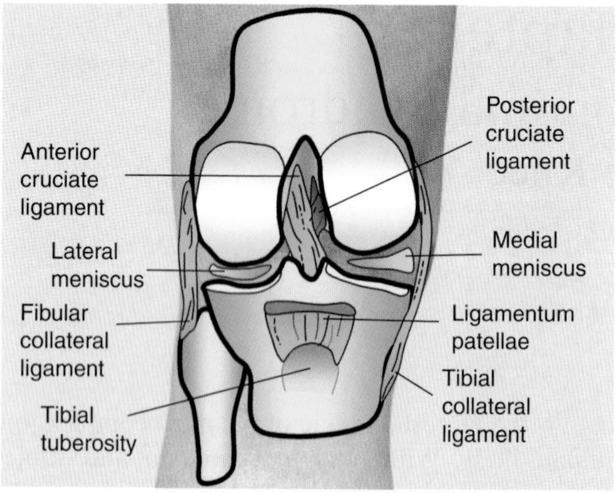

FIGURE 3.1 Bones and ligaments of the knee (*anterior view* – right knee)

the articular surfaces of the femur and tibia. On the anterior aspect of the distal femur, above the patella, it forms a large pouch, where articular fluid may accumulate. It is therefore an important area to include in the physical examination when looking for articular effusion or swelling (Fig. 3.2). The posterior face of the joint corresponds to the popliteal fossa. Here, the joint may communicate with the semimembranous bursa, forming a popliteal pouch. When this bursa is full of fluid, it forms a palpable, oval mass known as a Baker's cyst (Fig. 3.2).

The articular capsule is reinforced by resistant fibrous ligaments that join the femur to the tibia, forming the internal and external collateral knee ligaments. The cruciate ligaments are inside the joint.The anterior cruciate inserts above and behind on the internal face of the lateral femoral condyle and below and in front, on the anterior intercondyle area of the tibia. It therefore prevents the tibia from gliding anteriorly over the femur. The posterior cruciate is positioned the other way round and prevents the opposite movement. The muscles that operate the joint play an important role in its stability and, when strong, can partially compensate for weakness of the ligaments.

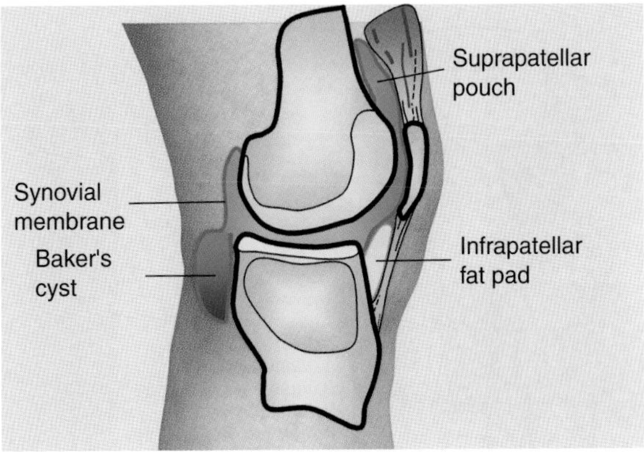

FIGURE 3.2 Synovial membrane of the knee and Baker's cyst (*medial view*)

The patella is suspended within the femoral quadriceps or patella tendon. The tendon inserts into its superior border and joins its inferior end to the tibial tuberosity. Two fibrous bands, the patellar retinacula, insert on each side of the patella and the corresponding faces of the femoral condyles, thus limiting the lateral mobility of the patella.

Load-bearing flexion and extension of the knee understandably cause firm compression of the patella against the femur. This may account for why patellofemoral osteoarthritis is more common in the obese and causes pain particularly when going up and down stairs. In cases of deviations of the patella (most often lateral) the pressure is exerted mainly on the condyle on that side, leading to rapid wearing of the cartilage and early osteoarthritis. Behind the patellar tendon is an fat pad known as Hoffa's fat pad, which may become inflamed.

The anterior face of the patella is covered by the prepatellar bursa, an occasional site of inflammation associated with repeated trauma ("clergyman's or housemaid's knee").

The knee is capable of flexion (about 135°), depending basically on the femoral biceps muscles, semitendinosus and semimembranosus, which are innervated by L5/S1. Extension

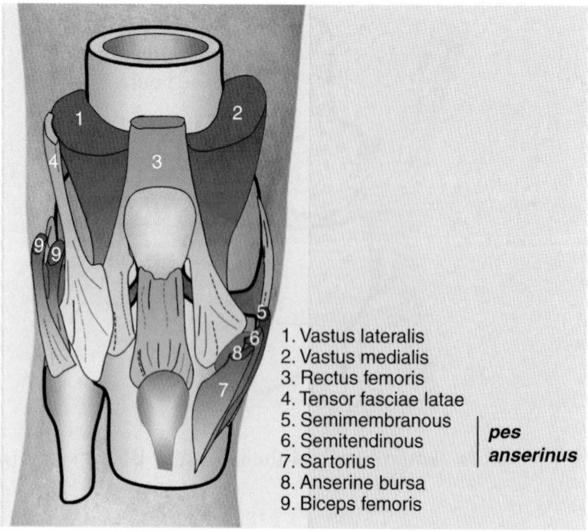

FIGURE 3.3 Muscle insertion around the knee (*anterior view* – right knee)

(0°) is the responsibility of the femoral quadriceps, which are innervated by L3/L4. There are also discreet rotation and anteroposterior gliding movements. Figure 3.3 shows the muscle insertions around the knee. The sensory innervation in this area is shown in Fig. 1.12.

A complex tendinous structure consisting of the tendons of the semitendinous and semimembranous muscles (coming from the iliac ischium) and the sartorius muscle (inserting superiorly in the anterosuperior iliac spine) inserts in the anteromedial face of the superiorend of the tibia. This structure is called the *pes anserinus*. Arranged deeply between these tendons is the anserine bursa. These structures are often the site of painful, incapacitating inflammation (Fig. 3.4).

Radiological Anatomy

In a weight-bearing anteroposteri or radiograph (Fig. 3.5), assess the size and regularity of the articular space and bone

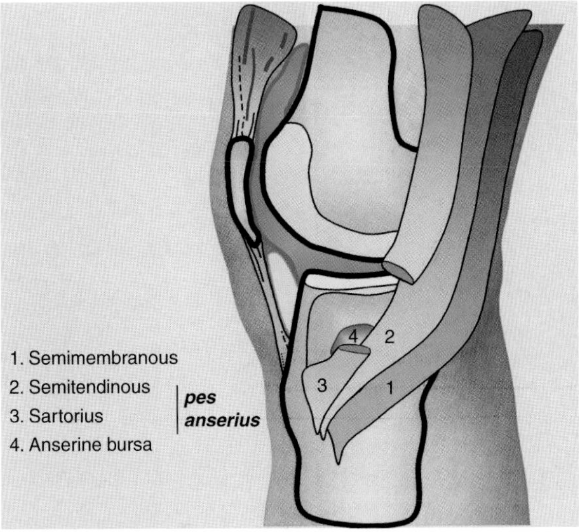

FIGURE 3.4 *Pes anserinus* and anserine bursa (*medial view* – right knee)

edges, inside and around the joint. Note the density of the subchondral bone. In profile, assess the same aspects and also the patellofemoral joint and tibial tuberosity.

Tangential projections of the patella at 30° of flexion (so-called "sky-line" views) compliment the study of the patell-ofemoral joint. Look for any external deviation of the patella, with sclerosis or a reduction in articular space.

Common Causes of Knee Pain

Osteoarthritis is the most common cause of knee pain. Periarticular lesions often occur in isolation or in association with joint disease (Table 3.1). Lesions of the ligaments and menisci are the main causes of knee pain in young people.

Chronic instability of the knee contributes to pain and aggra vation of the articular process.

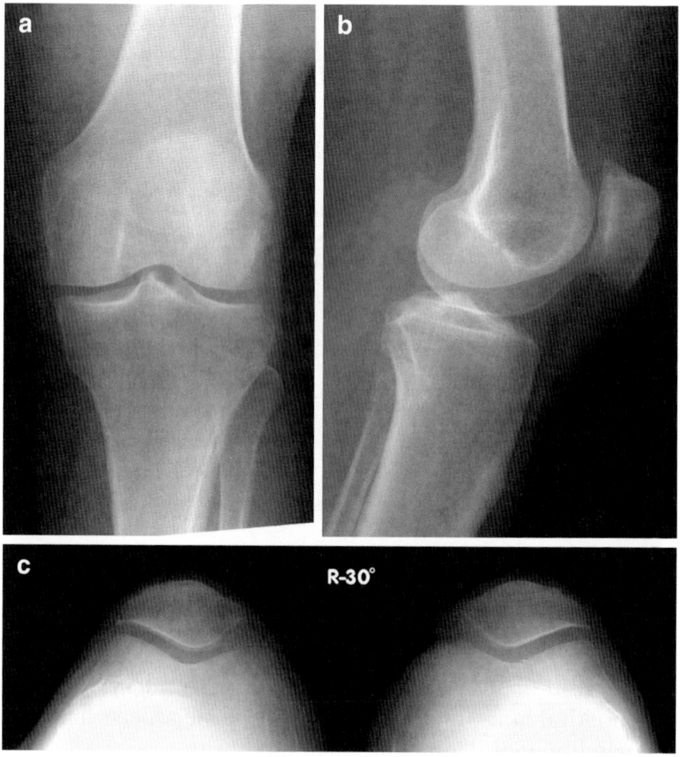

FIGURE 3.5 Radiographs of the knee. (**a**) Weight-bearing antero-posterior view. (**b**) Weight-bearing lateral view. (**c**) Skyline views of the patella (knee at 30° flexion)

The Enquiry

Age

The age of onset of a complaint gives us important clues as to the most probable diagnosis, as shown in Table 3.2

Rhythm of the Pain

In most cases the pain has a mechanical rhythm, associated with movement and relieved by rest. Exceptions are inflammatory

TABLE 3.1 The most common causes of knee pain

Etiology	Clinical clues
Osteoarthritis	Pain with mechanical rhythm Associated with obesity
Baker's cyst	Deep, moderate pain in the popliteal fossa Palpable cyst
Anserine bursitis/ tendonitis	Pain in the medial face of the knee Worse at night and with exercise Painful local palpation More frequent in obese women Often associated with knee joint disease
Lesions of the menisci	Recurring episodes of acute knee pain The knee locks or g ives way Predominant in young people and athletes
Instability of the knee	Unsteadiness and pain while walking Associated with trauma or chronic joint disease
Arthritis	Inflammatory knee pain Swelling, effusion or local heat
Referred pain	Diffuse painLocal examination inconclusive Pathology of the lumbar spine or hip
Anterior knee pain syndrome	Pain in the anterior face of the knee Variable rhythm, generally exacerbated by walking Examination generally inconclusive Predominant in young women

TABLE 3.2 Most common causes of knee pain, by age groups

Age group	Predominent causes
<15	Juvenile idiopathic arthritis Anterior knee pain syndrome Osgood-Schlatter's disease Hypermobility syndrome Hip diseases
10–30	Lesions of the meniscus Lesions of the ligaments Hypermobility syndrome Anterior knee pain syndrome
30–50	Lesions of the meniscus Lesions of the ligaments Anserine bursitis/tendonitis Patellofemoral osteoarthritis Baker's cyst Arthritis
>50	Osteoarthritis Baker's cyst Anserine bursitis/tendonitis

synovitis and anserine bursitis/tendonitis, in which it usually predominates at night or in the morning.

Onset and Progression

While the onset of pain related to osteoarthritis or Baker's cyst is usually insidious and progressive over months or years, pain caused by synovitis or bursitis/tendonitis appears in days or weeks. Ligamen tal lesions are very often acute and related to trauma.

Meniscal lesions in most patients are reflected by recurrent episodes of self-limiting pain often related to rotation on a load-bearing foot. Patients may say that their knee "gives way" (sudden weakness), or locks, i.e. the knee "gets stuck" in semi-flexion and then resumes movement after a while. These occurrences may be associated with transient swelling (a few days).

Signs of Inflammation

Descriptions by the patient of signs of inflammation of the knee (swelling, heat or redness) are highly suggestive of local inflammation. Note, however, that advanced osteoarthritis is often accompanied by indolent joint effusion. Meniscal lesions and chronic instability of the knee may also cause joint effusion.

Involvement of Other Joints

Many diseases of the knee are associated with similar developments in other joints, and their nature and location may help make the diagnosis. Knee osteoarthritis may be the first sign, but many patients also have mechanical back pain and degenerative change of the spine and, less commonly, the hip. Isolated acute or subacute synovitis of the knee should be considered septic until proven otherwise and referred urgently for the appropriate tests and treatment.

Remember that pain originating in the hip or the spine can radiate or even present as pain in the knee. It is important to examine these joints, especially if the examination of the knee is inconclusive.

Regional Examination

Inspection

Watch the way the patient walks when coming into the room or climbing onto the examination couch and check the alignment of the knees while the patient is standing. In normal conditions, the axis of the thigh with the lower leg forms an angle of about 5°. With an accentuation of this angle the patient is said to be knock-kneed (*genu valgus*). A deviation in the opposite direction is called *genu varus*, i.e. the patient is bowlegged, a very common deformity in patients with osteoarthritis.

Note the spontaneous position of the knees when the patient is lying down. Normally, the popliteal fossa is in contact with the couch. Any inability to do this indicates limited extension due either to pain or a fixed flexion deformity (Fig. 3.6).

Swelling or effusion of the knee is suggested by the disappearance of the bony contours (compare with the other knee – Fig. 3.6). A rounded swelling may be seen superior to the patella. These signs must be confirmed by palpation, however. Articular redness is rarely visible, even in cases of active arthritis. Skin redness overlying the joint is more commonly associated with septic, microcrystalline or reactive arthritis.

Look for signs of muscle wasting, which is common in chronic diseases of the knee and in neurological lesions (Fig. 3.7). The skin covering the anterior aspect of the knees is often the site of psoriasis.

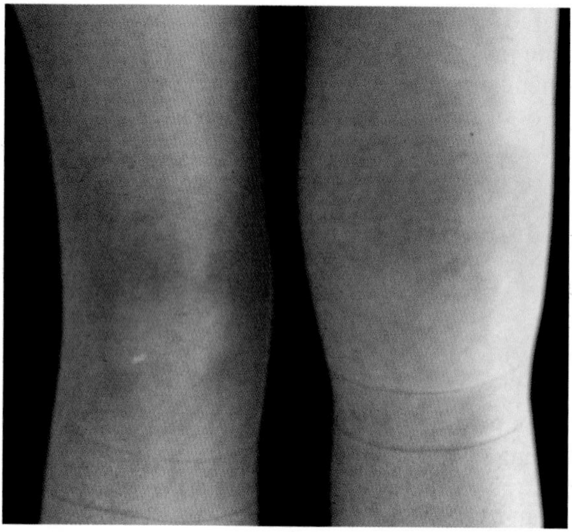

FIGURE 3.6 Swelling of the left knee: loss of bone contours and suprapatellar swelling. Patients usually keep the knee in flexion

Palpation

Feel the local temperature with the back of your hand and compare it to that of the thigh, lower leg and contralateral knee.

Palpate the joint space on either side of the patella (the articular space is at the level of the lower edge of the patella, when the patient is lying down). Synovial inflammation is suggested by the presence of elastic tissue covering the contour of the bone. Osteophytes, typical of osteoarthritis, feel like irregular bony spurs.

In synovitis, palpation usually causes pain along the whole articular space. In osteoarthritis, it is more typical to find various diffuse points of pain.

Also palpate the superior and inferior insertion points of the internal and external collateral ligaments to identify pain suggesting ligamentitis.

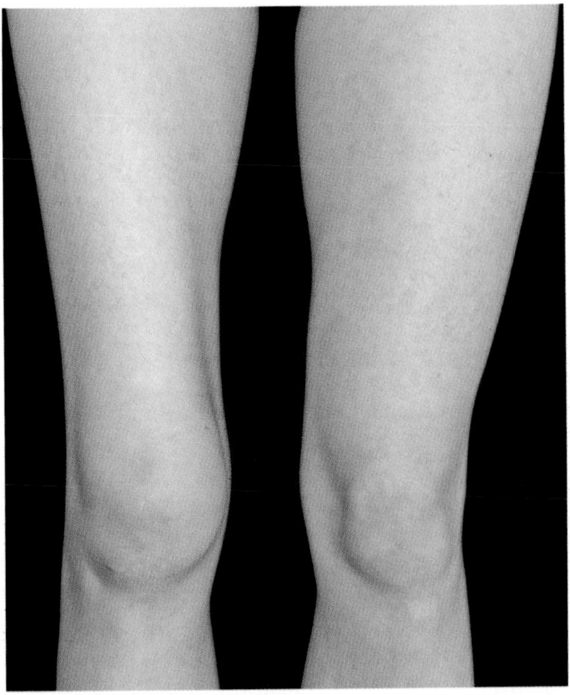

FIGURE 3.7 Muscle atrophy of the *right thigh* in association with ipsilateral knee arthritis

Palpate the *pes anserinus*, following it along the antero-medial face of the tibia and posteromedial edge of the knee. In cases of anserine bursitis/tendonitis, the patient will complain of intense pain (Fig. 3.8).

Looking for knee joint effusion

1. Firmly mold your palm to the upper part of the patient's knee, with the fold between your thumb

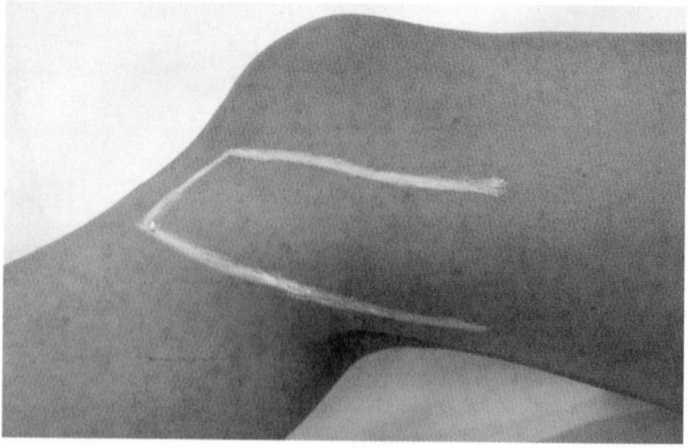

FIGURE 3.8 Area of tenderness associated with pes anserinus tendonitis (*Right knee*, medial aspect)

and index finger slightly above the upper edge of the patella. Squeeze the medial and lateral aspects of the knee with your fingers. This pushes the synovial fluid to the posterior face of the patella. With the thumb of your other hand, push the patella against the femur (Fig. 3.9). Normally, the patella should now be in contact with the femur and will not move. If there is effusion, there will be anteroposterior movement of the patella until it hits the femur (the "piano key sign").

Identifying joint effusion is a crucial aspect of the clinical assessment of the knee.

Note that the thumb must be in the centre of the patella, pushing it posteriorly. If it is not in the centre, the patella will swing and this can simulate effusion. A systematic check for this sign in all patients can do a lot to increase your sensitivity in detecting small volume effusions.

The following technique may be more effective for discrete effusions.

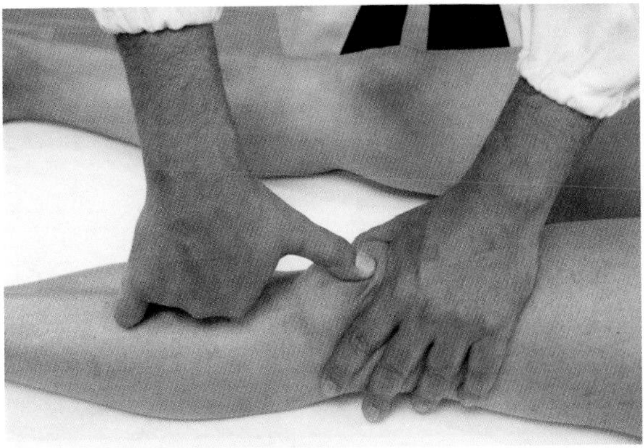

FIGURE 3.9 Looking for knee effusion (**1**). The *left hand* has been drawn down over the suprapatellar bursa forcing any fluid to accumulate under the patella. The *right thumb* is checking for fluctuation of the patella

Looking for knee joint effusion

2. Run the back of your hand firmly along the medial face of the knee so that any fluid accumulated there is pushed outward. Now run your hand along the outer face while watching the medial face of the knee carefully. Any effusion that is not under pressure will cause a small swelling to appear on the internal face of the knee, inside and above the patella (Fig. 3.10a and b).

Mobilization

Place one of your hands lightly on the knee. Hold the patient's leg with your other hand and induce maximum flexion and extension of the knee. Repeat these movements. The hand on the knee will detect any crepitus or snapping in the knee compartments. Osteoarthritis is accompanied by coarse crepitus. Light crepitus may also be perceptible in some other cases of arthritis.

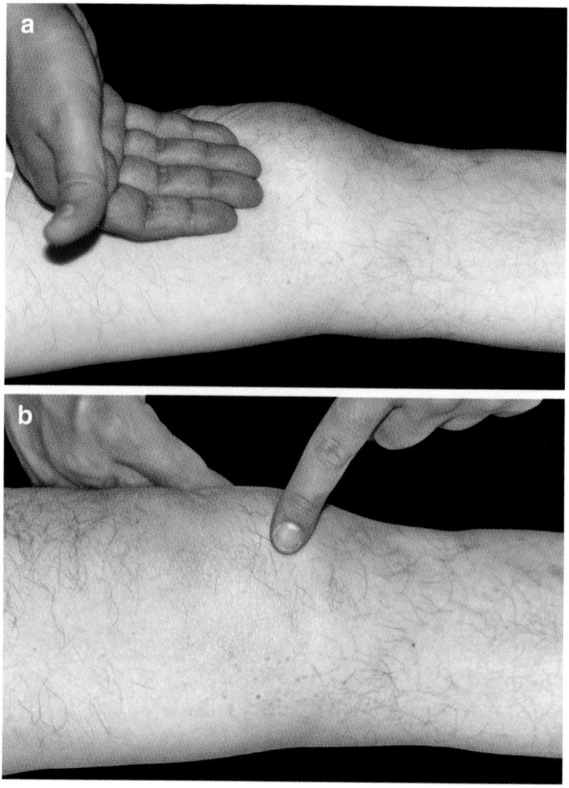

FIGURE 3.10 Looking for knee effusion (**2**). (**a**) Palpate firmly the medial aspect of the knee to move any effusion. (**b**) Now sweep the hand over the lateral aspect while examining the medial aspect: the relocation of a rounded swelling reveals the presence of moderate volume effusion

Note the range of movements. Both osteoarthritis and other arthritides may involve painful and/or structural limitation of mobility. Extension is normally 0°. In many normal young people, especially women, there may be hyperextension of up to 10°. Further than this, the movement is clearly excessive and may be part of the benign hypermobility syndrome.

Lesions of the posterior face of the patella (osteoarthritis, patellar chondromalacia) cause particularly intense pain when the patella is forced against the femur.

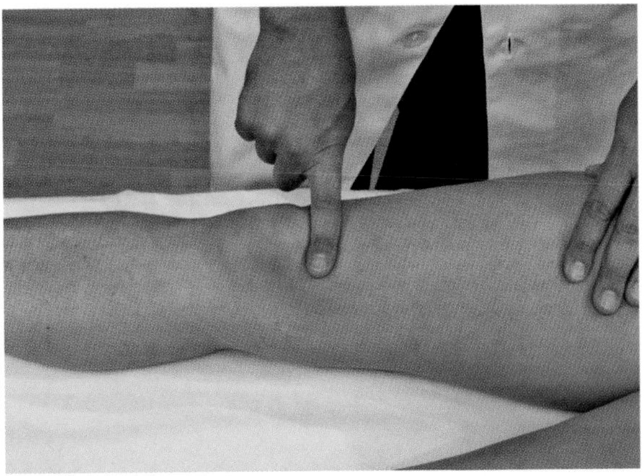

FIGURE 3.11 Patello-femoral maneuver. The index finger forces the 1. Collateral ligaments patella against the femur while the patients contracts the quadriceps, pulling the patella upwards

Examination of the patellofemoral joint
With the patient lying on their back and the knee relaxed and in extension, firmly press your index finger along the upper edge of the patella. Ask the patient to contract his quadriceps (or press his heel against the examining table) (Fig. 3.11). Intense pain when the patella is moved upward suggests a patellofemoral lesion.

Assessing joint stability.

1. Collateral ligaments
Firmly hold the knee by its internal face with one hand and the lower leg with the other, keeping the knee at about 30° flexion. Try to induce external deviation of the knee (genu varus).

Repeat the maneuver in the opposite direction (Fig. 3.12).

In the first maneuver, we test the competence of the external collateral ligament, while the second assesses the medial ligament. These maneuvers require training to avoid mistaking

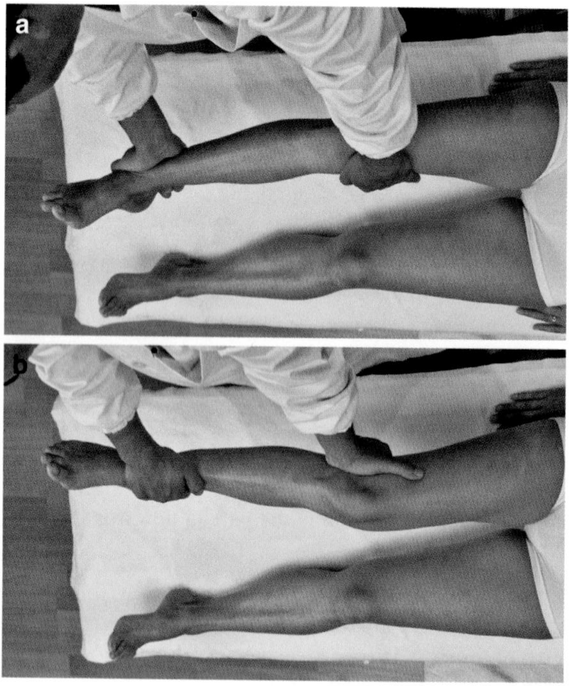

FIGURE 3.12 Checking knee stability. (**a**) Fibular collateral ligament. (**b**) Tibial collateral ligament (Vd. Explanations in text)

flexion of the knee for instability. Make sure that the movement is on the patient's coronal plane.

Instability of the lateral ligaments is very common in patients with advanced osteoarthritis, contributing decisively to the pain and progression of the degenerative process. This anomaly requires its own specific treatment. It may also be

2. Cruciate ligaments
Ask the patient to flex his knee to 90°, with his foot resting on the examination couch. Sit gently on the foot to immobilize it.

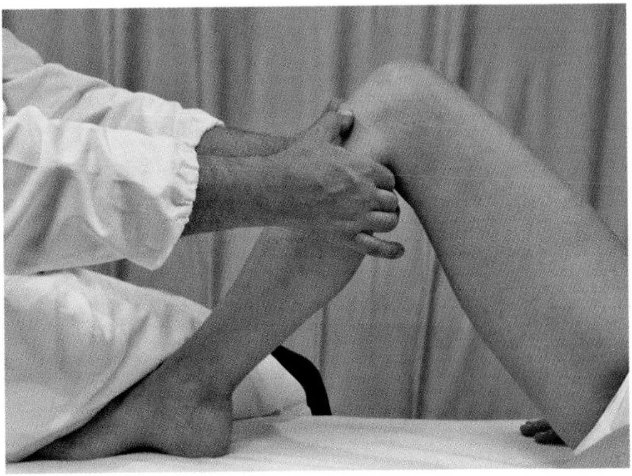

FIGURE 3.13 Assessing cruciate ligament integrity. With the knee flexed at 90° and the foot immobilized, the observer tests the antero-posterior mobility of the tibia on the femur

Firmly grasp the proximal end of the tibia with both hands. Try to induce anterior and then posterior movement (Fig. 3.13).

the result of trauma.

In these maneuvers we assess the dislocation of the tibia in relation to the femur. Excessive movement indicates impairmentof one of the cruciate ligaments. Rupture or laxicity of a cruciate ligament is usually secondary to trauma, but can also be found in patients with chronic arthritis of the knee.

1. McMurray's test
start with the knee flexed at 90°. One of your hands holds the patient's foot in internal rotation. The other holds the knee by its internal face pushing it outwards. While maintaining this pressure, induce repeated extension and flexion of the knee (Fig. 3.14a).

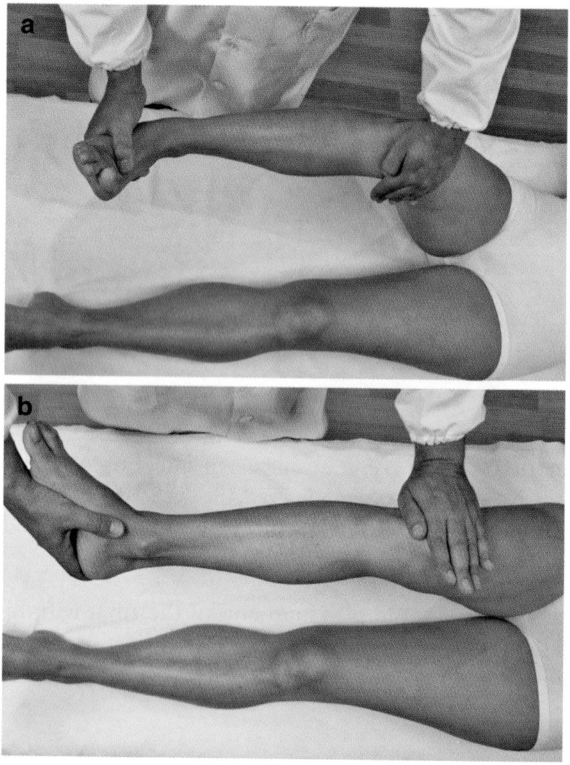

FIGURE 3.14 Assessing meniscus integrity. McMurray's test. (**a**) Medial meniscus. (**b**) Lateral meniscus (Vd. explanations in text)

Examining the menisci.

Pain in this maneuver indicates a lesion of the internal meniscus, which, with this method, is compressed between the femur and tibia. There is sometimes a snap or click in the joints, which reinforces the diagnosis.

Repeat the above maneuver, now rotating the foot outwards and pushing the knee inwards (Fig. 3.14b). This tests the external meniscus.

Typical Cases

3.A. Knee Pain (I)

Carlos Rodrigues was a cheerful 67-year old man who liked parties and outings. Unfortunately, he was no longer able to enjoy these pleasures in the same way because of growing pain in her knees seriously limiting her ability to walk. The pain was typically mechanical, appearing with exercise, especially walking and climbing stairs, and disappearing completely while lying down. It was particularly intense when he got up and walked after sitting for some time. This caused him to say initially that it was worse with rest! He described intense morning and post-rest stiffness lasting 5–10 minutes, known as "gelling."

The pain had begun 5 or 6 years before and worsened progressively. Anti-inflammatories and local heat were increasingly ineffective. He complained of chronic, mechanical backache, which was reasonably controlled. He was being treated for hypertension and non-insulin dependent diabetes. He had a history of gastritis and anemia.

What possible causes are you thinking of?
Program the clinical examination in your mind.

On clinical examination we found the patient limped and was clearly bowlegged (Fig. 3.15). He was plainly obese (weight 72 kg, height 1,47 m).

Examination of the lumbar spine showed a painful reduction in mobility on flexion and extension. The hip joints were normal. The knees presented about 10° genu varus. Inspection suggested deformation of the joint. Palpation showed no increase in local temperature. We noted pain and osteophytes on palpation of the medial joint space bilaterally and discreet joint effusion on the right. Palpation of the pes anserinus was painless. The external collateral ligament was impaired bilaterally. Mobilization revealed a painful reduction in flexion to about 90° on the right and 80° on the left with accentuated crepitus of the patella and internal compartment.

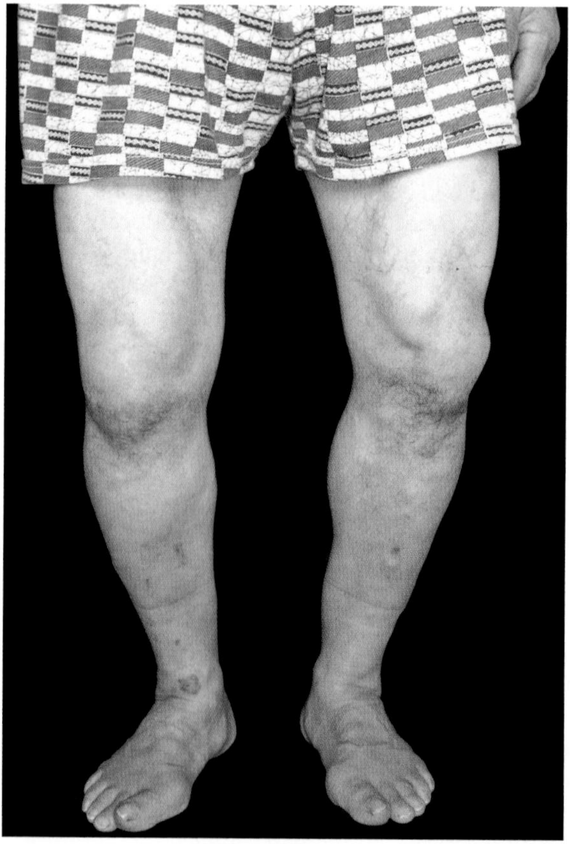

FIGURE 3.15 Clinical case "Knee pain (I)." Note the distance between the knees while the patient stands – *Genu varum*

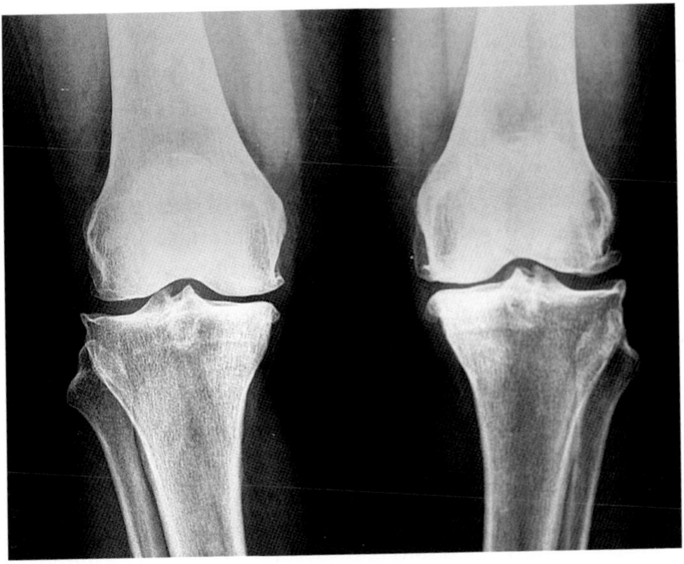

FIGURE 3.16 Knee X-rays. Clinical case "Knee pain (I)"

Briefly summarize the main problems.[1]

What is your diagnosis?

Were diagnostic tests necessary? What would you expect from them?

What treatment would you recommend?

We concluded that the patient had advanced osteoarthritis, with probable involvement of the knees and lumbar spine. An x-ray of the knees confirmed this diagnosis (Fig. 3.16). We also requested a full blood count and kidney function tests to monitor the treatment.

We explained the situation to the patient, stressing its etiological relationship with his obesity and recommending a "radical" change in his eating habits. We suggested and explained some exercises for strengthening the quadriceps and ischiotibial muscles, to be done twice a day.

---

[1]Progressive-onset knee pain and mechanical backache in an obese middle-aged man. Objective alterations of a degenerative nature. *Genu varus*.

Osteoarthritis of the Knee

Main Points

It is very common in patients over 60 years of age although it may appear before.

More common in women.

Its starts insidiously and may get progressively worse.

It causes typically mechanical pain, though there may be periods of inflammatory exacerbation, with effusion and nocturnal pain.

Clinical examination may reveal crepitus, painful limitation of mobility and osteophyte excrescences. Joint effusion may be present.

There is often instability of the knee ligaments, which exacerbates the situation.

It most commonly affects the medial tibiofemoral compartment and the patellofemoral joints.

It is closely related to being overweight. Local trauma or inflammation and hard physical labor are other risk factors.

X-ray changes are typical of osteoarthritis.

The treatment of osteoarthritis is described in Chap. 16.

Unfortunately, the analgesic that we would have preferred to prevent the side effects of the anti-inflammatories,[2] had already proved ineffective. We therefore prescribed an anti-inflammatory drug combined with a proton-pump inhibitor and advised a regular monitoring of his blood pressure. We suggested local heat and massages with a topical anti-inflammatory during flare-ups. Mr. Rodrigues refused to use a stick. We may have to consider a joint prosthesis depending on his progress.

Give a brief description of the problem.[3]

What is the most probable diagnosis?

---

[2]What risk factors for anti-inflammatories can you identify in this patient? Aged over 65, history of gastritis, anemia and hypertension.

[3]Acute, post-infectious monoarthritis in a young woman.

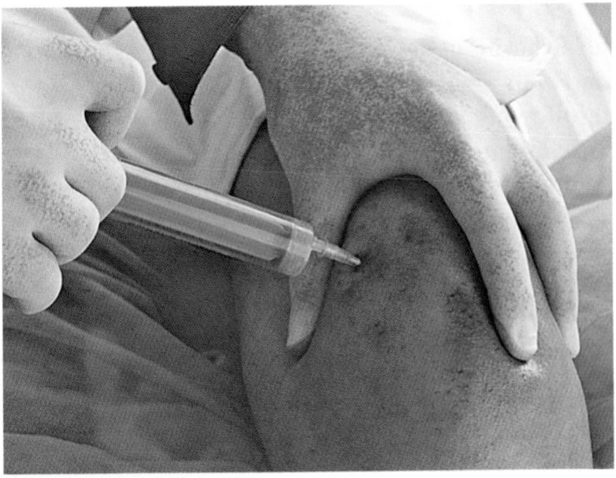

FIGURE 3.17 Clinical case "Knee pain (II)." Arthrocentesis revealed a clowdy synovial fluid

Typical Cases
3.B. Knee Pain (Ii)
Joana Castelão, a 21-year old student, came to the emergency department because of intense pain in her left knee that had begun 2 days before and rapidly become incapacitating. Her knee was hot, swollen and slightly red. Palpation was painful all around the joint and there was a large, tense effusion (Fig. 3.6). Her axillary temperature was 38.2°C.

Three weeks earlier she had gone on a school trip, and she and other members of the group had developed febrile gastroenteritis, for which they had been treated successfully with antibiotics.

How would you proceed in terms of additional investigation?

There could be no doubt as to the diagnosis of acute arthritis. Her history of infection strongly suggested post-dysenteric reactive arthritis or, less likely, septic arthritis.

Acute Synovitis of the Knee

Main Points

The following indicate an acute synovitis[4] of the knee:

- Inflammatory pain
- Synovial swelling and/or joint effusion
- Local heat
- The diagnosis is clinical: it only requires laboratory tests for etiological investigation

It often appears in a context of poly or oligoarthritis. It is the joint most often affected by idiopathic juvenile arthritis.

Monoarthritis of the knee should be considered infectious until proven otherwise.Reactive arthritis and microcrystalline arthritis are other possibilities. It is essential to aspirate and examine synovial fluid.

In cases of unexplained monoarthritis consider the possibility of algodystrophy.

Treatment depends on the clinical and etiological context and should always be guided by specialists.

A stool culture conducted in hospital was negative. Serological studies revealed high levels of anti-Salmonella typhi antibodies. Her sedimentation rate was 56 mm in the first hour. We aspirated the joint (Fig. 3.17) and the fluid had the expected inflammatory characteristics: cloudy, low viscosity, and 18,000 leukocytes per mm3 (80% neutrophils). A bacteriological examination and crystal test were negative.

These findings were consistent with a diagnosis of **reactive arthritis**.

What treatment would you suggest?

We administered an intra-articular injection of 40 mg triamcinolone hexacetonide, which rapidly alleviated the symptoms. There were no recurrences in the following three months.

---

[4]By "synovitis" we understand "inflammatory arthritis" as opposed to osteoarthritis.

We explained the nature of the disease, emphasizing that it generally cleared up completely. There was, however, still a risk of recurrence due to reinfection, as the previous episode had demonstrated a genetic predisposition to this type of reaction.

Typical Cases
3.C. Knee Pain (III)
Maria Rosa had already been treated at our clinic for moderate osteoarthritis of the knees for several years. She called and asked for an emergency appointment because the pain had become worse 2 weeks previously. She also had pain at night now, especially in her right knee, which kept her awake. The pain was more intense lying on her side. Normally morning stiffness was negligible but now it lasted about 30 minutes. Her usual simple analgesics were no longer effective and her knee was more swollen.

Examination of her right knee showed a discreet increase in skin temperature, accompanied by pain along the joint space and large effusion. Palpation of the pes anserinus caused extreme pain as far as the posterosuperior edge of the medial femoral condyle.

How would you explain this condition?
What treatment would you recommend?

We concluded that our patient was suffering an **inflammatory flare of her knee osteoarthritis**, which was now associated with **anserine tendonitis**.

We recommended partial rest and temporarily replaced the simple analgesics by a full dose of anti-inflammatories. We added a topical anti-inflammatory to be applied to the medial knee three times a day. Three weeks later she was much better. The stiffness and the articular effusion had gone. Although it was not too bad, she still had some pain on lying down and with some movements. A local examination confirmed the persistence of the anserine tendonitis, though the painful area was much smaller. We administered a local injection of a mixture of local anesthetic and glucocorticoid, which relieved the pain. The patient went back to her normal analgesic and was reminded to do the muscle-strengthening exercises we had advised.

Anserine Bursitis/Tendonitis

Main Points

It is a very common cause of pain, especially in obese middle-aged women.

It appears most often as an aggravation of a known joint disease, but may occur in isolation.

The pain predominates on the medial aspect of the knee and is aggravated by sudden movements of the lower limbs and lying on the side.

Pain on palpation is the key to the diagnosis.

Treatment is based on rest and the application of local anti-inflammatories.

In stubborn cases, provided that the painful area is not too large, a local injection may be effective.

Physiotherapy can be used in difficult cases.

In exceptional cases, surgery may be necessary.

Typical Cases

3.D. Knee Pain (IV)

Madalena Rosado, a 21-year old student, came to the clinic because of pain in her left knee. It had first occurred about 8 years before when she was doing ballet, sometimes forcing her to wear an elastic bandage. The pain was intermittent, appearing suddenly and lasting 2 or 3 days, sometimes with joint swelling. After giving up her favorite physical activity, it occurred less frequently, when she was getting into or out of a car, for example. She felt discomfort in her knees after sitting for a long time. When asked, she described one or two episodes when her knee "gave way," but she denied that it locked.

A more detailed enquiry revealed that she also had transient pain in other joints, like her wrists and shoulders though it was rare. She had a history of several "sprains," which she attributed to ballet.

General examination showed she had great articular flexibility and agility (she placed her palms on the floor with ease, keeping straight legs). Examination of the knees found no deviations, swelling, pain, crepitus or limited mobility. We noticed knee hyperextension of about 20° and appreciable instability of the collateral ligaments. The cruciates were competent.

What possible explanations were there for this situation?

Was there some pathology underlying the more dispersed pain?

How would you complete the physical examination?

The maneuvers for assessing the left internal meniscus caused intense pain, while the others were normal.

We conducted a specific examination for hypermobility of other joints. The patient had no trouble in putting her palms on the floor, and there was about 15° hyperextension of the elbows. We could get her thumb to touch her forearm and the fifth metacarpophalangeal joint easily achieved 90° extension (Fig. 3.18). The skin was normal.

Our patient very probably had a **lesion of the internal meniscus** of the left knee in association with the benign **hypermobility syndrome**, which was confirmed by the above criteria. This condition probably played an important role in the lesion

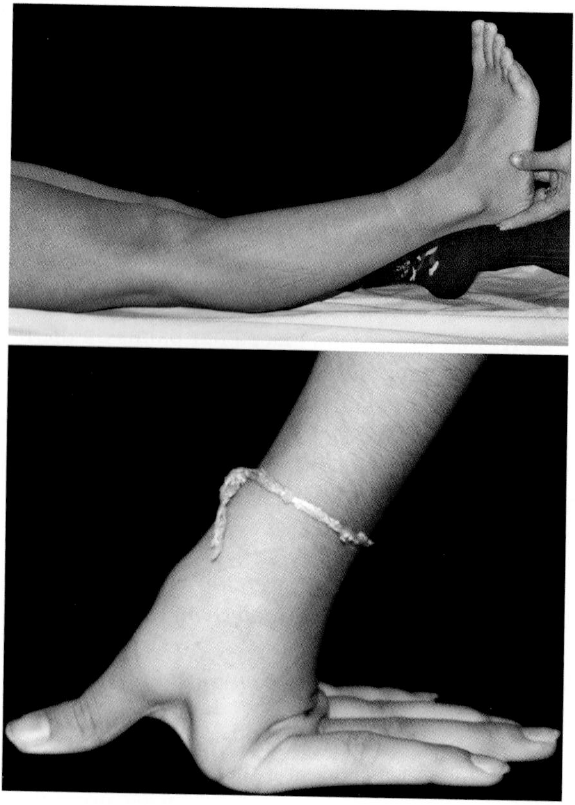

FIGURE 3.18 Clinical case "Knee pain (**IV**)." Two of the criteria for hypermobility syndrome: hyperextension of knee and metacarpophalangeal joints

of the left internal meniscus and *explained the intermittent, migratory pain as well as the tendency to suffer sprains.*

We explained the situation to the patient, stressing that the hypermobility that had been so useful in ballet facilitated repeated articular subluxations with transient pain in several joints. It could also have contributed to the lesion of the meniscus. We reassured her about the prognosis and made it clear that it was not the polyarticular inflammatory disease that she feared. We suggested that the physical exercise, which she continued to do, should be devoted to strengthening her muscles, though she should avoid extreme range of joint movements. Elastic bandages on the most susceptible joints might also be useful as well as specific exercises to strengthen supporting muscles.

Where the meniscus was concerned, we agreed that it was not serious enough for surgery. We therefore did not request an MRI at this stage, which is the best way of formally diagnosing this condition.

Meniscal Lesions

Main Points

They occur mainly in young individuals, and especially in athletes. They can contribute considerably to pain and disability in chronic knee conditions.

They cause acute-onset, recurring pain, with spontaneous recovery. With time, the pain becomes more persistent.

It may be accompanied by joint effusion during flares.

Many patients describe their knee "giving way" (sudden weakness) or locking (the knee gets stuck in semi-flexion, recovering gradually and painfully to normal mobility).

There may be pain on deep palpation of the anterior part of the joint space, on either side of the patellar tendon. McMurray's test is essential in confirming a suspected diagnosis.

Sports, instability of the knee and hypermobility syndrome are important risk factors.

Tolerable cases do not require diagnostic tests and are treated with measures to strengthen the muscles and elastic supports.

Persistent or incapacitating pain warrants confirmation by MRI, in preparation for a meniscectomy.

Meniscectomy increases the risk of later development of osteoarthritis, and should not be undertaken lightly.

Hypermobility Syndrome

Main Points

This condition consists of generalized laxity of the ligaments and skin in otherwise healthy people. It may cause recurring episodes of transient pain in several joints, with no signs of inflammation or criteria for fibromyalgia.

The knees (patella), shoulders, and tibiotarsal, metacarpophalangeal and temporomandibular joints are often affected.

The repeated episodes favor the occurrence of secondary osteoarthritis.

The diagnosis is based on the patient's ability to carry out a number of "exaggerated" movements. Give one point to each sign:

- Passive extension of the fifth MCP > 90°
- Passive contact of the thumb with the forearm
- Hyperextension of the elbow > 0°
- Hyperextension of the knee > 0°
- Touching the floor with the palms with the knees in extension

Right and left 1 point for each side

Diagnosis: 4 or more points + joint pain for more than three months in four or more joints.

Other syndromes involving hypermobility must be excluded, like Ehlers-Danlos syndrome, Marfan's syndrome and osteogenesis imperfecta.

Treatment is conservative, without medication.

Typical Cases

3.E. Knee Pain(V)

A colleague from vascular surgery referred 56-year old Alberto Falcão to us. He had come to the emergency department because of suspected deep vein thrombosis in the right leg. The Echo-Doppler was negative, however. Was there a rheumatologic cause?

The patient believed he had knee osteoarthritis, for which his GP had prescribed anti-inflammatory analgesia. His symptoms were compatible with this diagnosis: typically mechanical, slowly progressive pain. Sometimes, the joint would swell, forming a painful "lump" at the back of the knee, which made walking difficult. The week before, he had taken a long walk during which he had intense pain in the right calf, which prevented him from continuing. The next day, the pain was even worse and accompanied by accentuated swelling of the whole leg below the knee.

Baker's Cyst

Main Points

This is the collection of synovial fluid at the semimembranous bursa, which communicates with the knee joint forming a cul-de-sac.

It can appear in isolation, but usually accompanies diseases of the knee.

It can cause pain and discomfort in the popliteal fossa, where it is palpable (and sometimes visible) as an ovalswelling in the superomedial part of the popliteal fossa.

An ultrasound scan is a sensitive method of confirming the diagnosis.

If the patient is symptomatic, it may require ultrasound-guided drainage with a large needle, followed by infiltration or even surgery.

A ruptured Baker's cyst causes symptoms similar to deep vein thrombosis and may, rarely, develop into compartmental syndrome with edema, ischemia and muscular necrosis.

In a rupture, the echo-doppler may show alterations compatible with vein thrombosis. Ultrasound and arthrography of the knee are the best examinations, though it may be necessary to conduct a venography to exclude the differential diagnosis.

Give a brief description of this condition.[5]
What are the possible diagnoses at this stage?

An examination of the knees confirmed the presence of coarse crepitus and palpable osteophytes, with slight bilateral limitation of extension. On the left, there was clearly a large Baker's cyst, but not on the right. There was no joint effusion. Palpation of the right calf was extremely painful and there was accentuated edema and pitting in the median and lower third of the leg. Hommans' sign was positive (passive dorsiflexion of the foot caused pain in the calf). Everything pointed to vein thrombosis except the Doppler…

How would you explain the situation?
Would you request any diagnostic tests?

We asked for an ultrasound scan of the knees and calf, which confirmed bilateral Baker's cysts. In the right calf, there was a layer of liquid outside the muscles suggesting a probable rupture of the Baker's cyst on that side. The echo-Doppler showed diffuse vascular compression caused by edema of the gastrocnemius, but no vein thrombosis. We avoided ordering an arthrography of the knee, as there is usually clear loss of the contrast agent into the lower leg muscles.

We admitted the patient for rest, articular injection of corticosteroids and physical therapy, for rapid relief of the symptoms and to prevent the (real) risk of deep vein thrombosis induced by muscular edema in reaction to the synovial fluid.

Symptoms suggesting deep vein thrombosis of the calf in a patient with a disease of the knee should always raise the possibility of rupture of a Baker's cyst. They may be clinically indistinguishable!

---

[5]Condition suggesting deep vein thrombosis in a patient with knee osteoarthritis.

Special Situations

Anterior Knee Pain Syndrome

This is an ill-defined condition affecting mainly young women. It is characterized by pain in the anterior aspect of the knee, growing progressively worse and having a variable relation to movement, rest and cold weather. The clinical examination is perfectly normal. Diagnostic tests, including arthroscopy, are also normal.

In some cases, the pain seems to be caused by a synovial plica that can insinuate itself between the patella and the femur, where it is compressed and occasionally causes intra-articular hemorrhage. The diagnosis is not evident even on MRI, and is only possible after an arthroscopy, though even then there are limitations.

In other situations there is pain when applying pressure on the medial or lateral border of the patella, suggesting inflammation of the alae of the patella, which it is impossible to confirm.

Chondromalacia patella consists of a softening of the posterior cartilage of the patella. It causes mechanical pain, particularly exacerbated by going up or down stairs and generally beginning in adolescence. The usual maneuvers for this joint cause pain. Only arthroscopy can confirm the diagnosis. It has no specific treatment, but tends to resolve spontaneously after the age of 20–25.

A relatively common condition is lateral deviation of the patella. It is caused by an increase in the Q angle (> 20° - Fig. 3.19), which results in accentuated compression of the patella against the lateral condyle of the femur, with patellar pain and accelerated wear, leading ultimately to osteoarthritis. Clinical suspicion of this condition should lead to a skyline film of the patella with the knee flexed at 30°. An outward deviation of the patella in relation to the intercondylar axis, sometimes already associated with a reduction in joint space or subchondral sclerosis, strengthens the diagnosis. Treatment involves physiotherapy exercises to strengthen the vastus

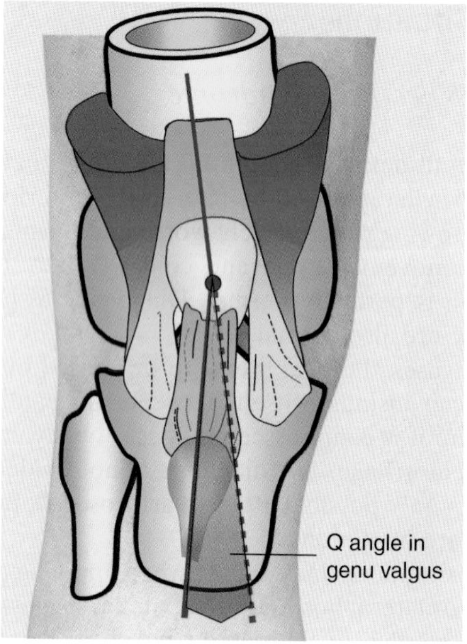

FIGURE 3.19 Positioning of the patella: Q angle in genu valgus

medialis. It is, however, sometimes associated with a retraction of the internal ala of the patella. Surgical correction of this anomaly is simple and often relieves the symptoms. It is important to note, however, that it is not known whether this procedure reduces or increases the risk of patellofemoral osteoarthritis in the long term.

In spite of the above, a high percentage of cases of anterior knee pain persist in the medium term with no precise diagnosis and therefore without specific treatment. Analgesics or anti-inflammatories are used as needed. Muscle-strengthening exercises for the quadriceps and distension of the ischiotibials are often useful. The use of an elastic knee band has contradictory results from one case to another. Patients should avoid high heels as they increase the pressure of the patella against the femur. These conditions tend to resolve spontaneously by the age of 25–30.

Osteochondritis Dissecans

This is a relatively rare cause of knee pain and is found in young men. A fragment of cartilage and subchondral bone detaches itself from the rest of the bone and becomes an intra-articular foreign body causing pain and recurrent locking of the knee joint.

Plain films show a radiolucent area where the fragment has separated. MRI is required to demonstrate intra-articular loose body. Treatment is surgical.

Algodystrophy

This is a localized vasomotor disturbance causing local pain, swelling, redness and heat, simulating monoarthritis. It often follows trauma but this is not always apparent in the history. See Chap. 4 for a more detailed description.

Osgood-Schlatter's Disease and Referred Pain

Particularly in children, pain in the knee may be caused by diseases of the hip. Osgood-Schlatter's disease typically presents in adolescence and consists of osteitis and enthesitis of the inferior insertion of the patellar tendon into the tibial tuberosity. It causes pain, which is aggravated by walking. Both Osgood-Schlatter's and referred knee pain are explained in more detail in Chap. 28.

Diagnostic Tests

As the knee joint is superficial, it lends itself to a detailed, highly informative clinical examination. This limits the need for diagnostic tests to situations in which we wish to assess the degree of structural alteration in the joint or evaluate theaetiology of arthritis.

Imaging

A plain film of the knees is indicated whenever clinical examination suggests an unexplained articular problem. It should be conducted with the patient standing, weight-bearing and is usually from two angles. Under these circumstances, the distance between the bones is a good indication of the thickness of the articular cartilage. In osteoarthritis, a sharpening of the tibial spines is one of the earliest signs. Loss of articular space tends to be asymmetrical, more pronounced in the medial compartment. Whether this is due to pre-existing genu varum or whether this develops secondary to disease, is the subject of current studies. Subchondral sclerosis, the formation of cysts and osteophytosis become more pronounced over time (Fig. 3.20).

The study of the patellofemoral joint requires a profile of the knee and a skyline view at 30° flexion.

In the inflammatory arthritides, radiological changes appear late. As in osteoarthritis, there is loss of joint space reflecting cartilage loss, which may be more diffuse. It is usually accompanied by periarticular osteopenia (unlike subchondral sclerosis). Erosions are rarely visible (Fig. 3.21).

Ultrasound scans are particularly useful in identifying small Baker's cysts (Fig. 3.22). Ultrasound scans are frequently normal in clinically manifest anserine bursitis/tendonitis. Ultrasound is not a good method for studying the menisci, MRI is much better.

An MRI is only justified when an unexplained, incapacitating situation justifies consideration of surgery.

Other Tests

Any synovial fluid aspirated from the knee should be sent for testing, even if the etiological diagnosis has already been clearly established as secondary infection is always a possibility. This test is clearly mandatory and urgent in the case of monoarthritis of the knee. A total and differential cell count is always important, to distinguish between a mechanical and an inflammatory process. Testing for crystals and bacteriological

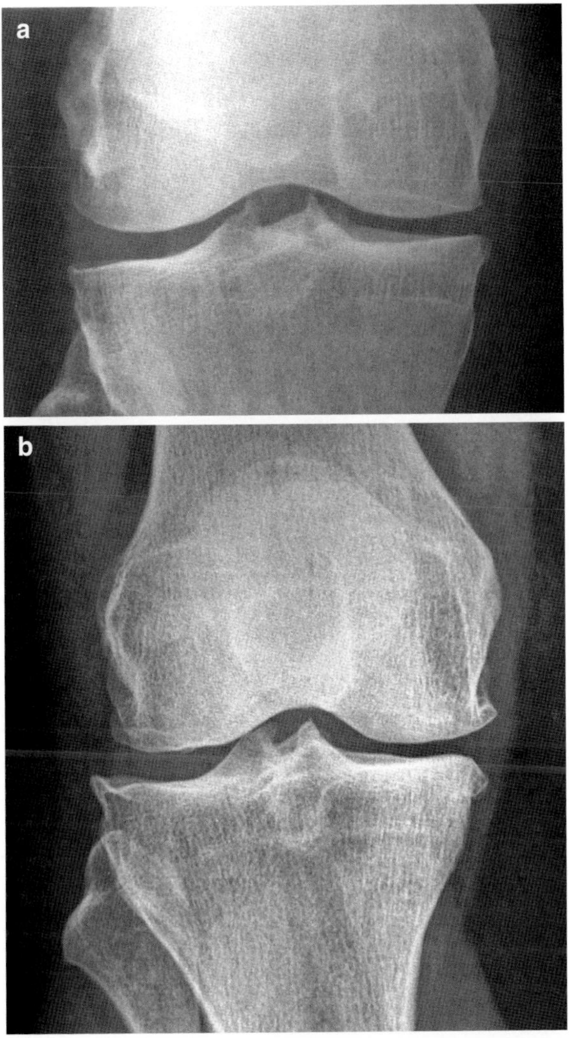

FIGURE 3.20 Radiological features of osteoarthritis. (**a**) Sharpening of the tibial spines is one of the earlier signs. (**b**) Joint space loss and osteophyte formation start at early stages of the disease. (**c**) Joint space loss tends to be assymetrical. Subchondral sclerosis, geodes and osteophytes become more prominent with time. Please note that a marginal osteophytes can simulate an erosion immediately above or below. (**d**) The patello-femoral joint is assessed with the lateral (and skyline) views

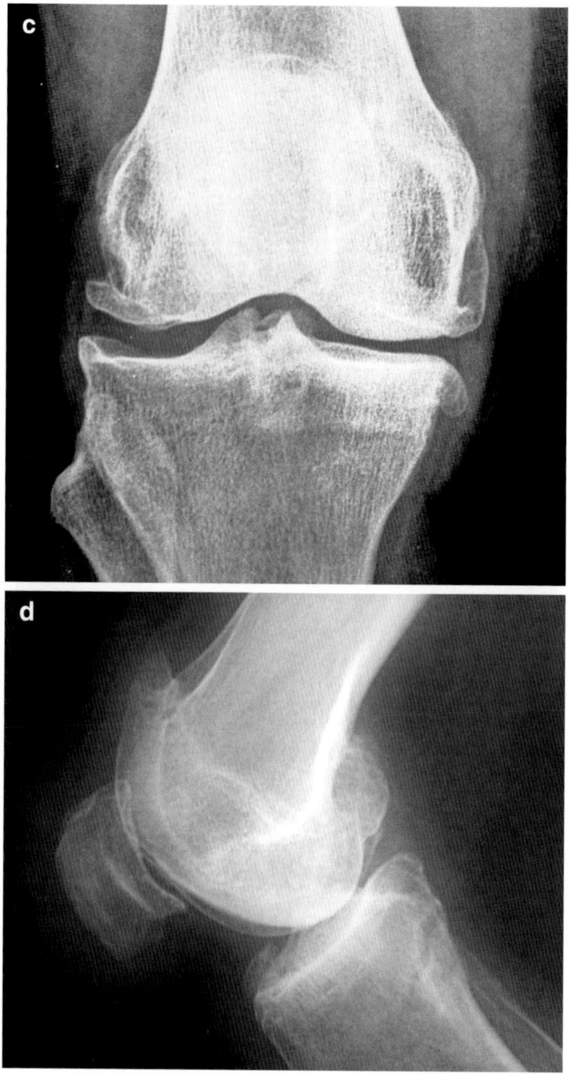

FIGURE 3.20 (continued)

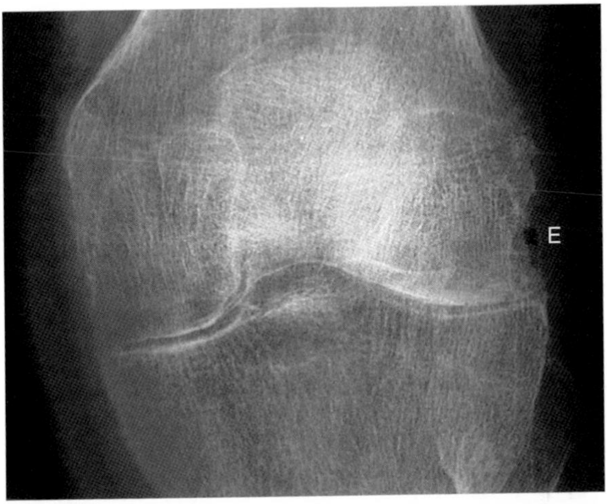

FIGURE 3.21 Knee X-rays in advanced inflammatory arthritis. Note that joint space loss is homogeneous and symmetrical. There is subchondral osteopenia (as opposed to sclerosis) and erosions can be present (E)

culture are indicated whenever clinical assessment admits the possibility of microcrystalline or septic arthritis.

Diagnostic arthroscopy may be necessary in complex cases.

Blood and urine tests will be guided by the clinical context,in an appropriate differential diagnosis strategy.

When Should the Patient be Referred to a Specialist?

Whenever there is arthritis of unknown cause.

When the degree of pain or disability is not explained by the clinical examination and plain films. When there is effusion, if the study of synovial fluid is deemed important for differential diagnosis (e.g. in the suspicion of gout).

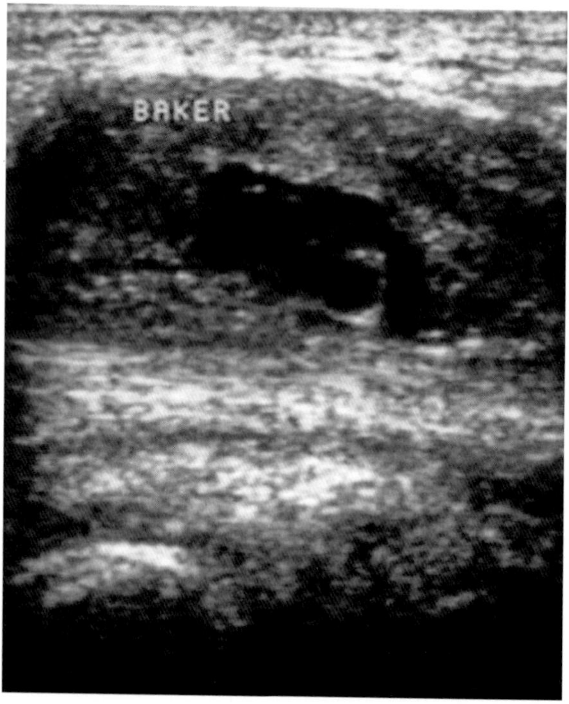

FIGURE 3.22 Baker's cyst revealed by ultrasonography of the popliteal area

In cases of meniscal lesions or bursitis/tendonitis that are resistant to standard treatment. In severe functional disability, with significant limitation of mobility (physiotherapy). In acute ruptures of the ligaments or chronic, accentuated joint instability (orthopedics). In osteoarthritis, whenever doubts persist as to the diagnosis (rheumatology) or if surgery is indicated (orthopedics).

Chapter 4
Regional Syndromes
The Foot and Ankle

Pain in the foot and ankle is a very common reason for a visit to the doctor. It can cause considerable suffering and disability, as walking is one of the activities that most influences a person's functional capacity and quality of life. Anatomically speaking, the foot combines great strength with a remarkable adaptability. A diagnosis is usually quite clear after a well focused enquiry and careful clinical examination, opening the way to successful treatment.

Functional Anatomy

The ankle and foot constitute a highly complex structure which lends itself to remarkable versatility and strength. The main function of the foot and ankle is to support the body's weight and distribute it throughout the weight-bearing structure as well as generating a spring effect to facilitate locomotion. At the same time, the structure is able to adapt itself to irregular surfaces and constant variations in the mechanical requirements that are imposed upon it.

The ankle and foot are made up of three functional units (Fig. 4.1):

a) The **hindfoot**, consisting of the distal extremities of the tibia and fibula, the talus and calcaneus and their joints and ligaments
b) The midfoot or **tarsus**, consisting of five small bones
c) The **forefoot**, consisting of the metatarsals, proximal, medial and distal phalanges, and their joints

J.A.P. da Silva, A.D. Woolf, *Rheumatology of the Lower Limbs in Clinical Practice*, DOI 10.1007/978-1-4471-2253-1_4,

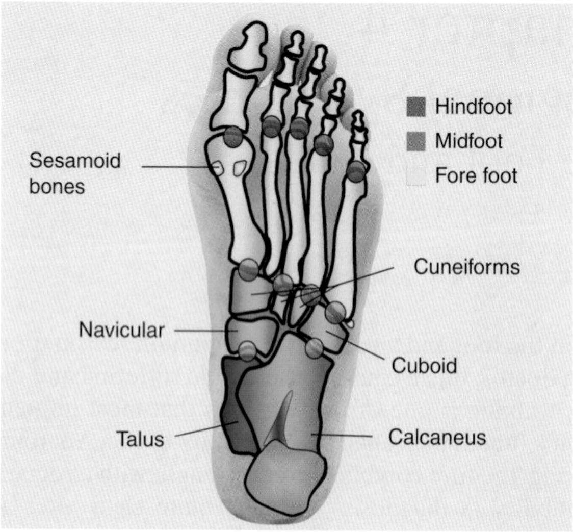

FIGURE 4.1 Bones and joints of the ankle and foot. Functional units

The joints of the hindfoot are stabilized by a complex set of ligaments (Fig. 4.2). These ligaments, especially those of the ankle joint, are frequently the site of traumatic lesions, with sprains or ruptures, which may result in chronic articular instability.

The Arches of the Foot

Under normal conditions, the bony structure is kept arched, a shape essential for distributing loads and achieving the spring effect. The anteroposterior arch is more accentuated in the medial aspect of the foot. It is maintained both by the form of the bones and by the ligaments that provide both resistance and elasticity (Fig. 4.2). The most superficial of these ligaments is the plantar fascia, a strong, fibrous band that connects the lower edge of the calcaneus to the transverse ligament of the metatarsals (under their distal extremities).

This fascia is understandably exposed to very powerful distending forces and to repeated trauma by compression,

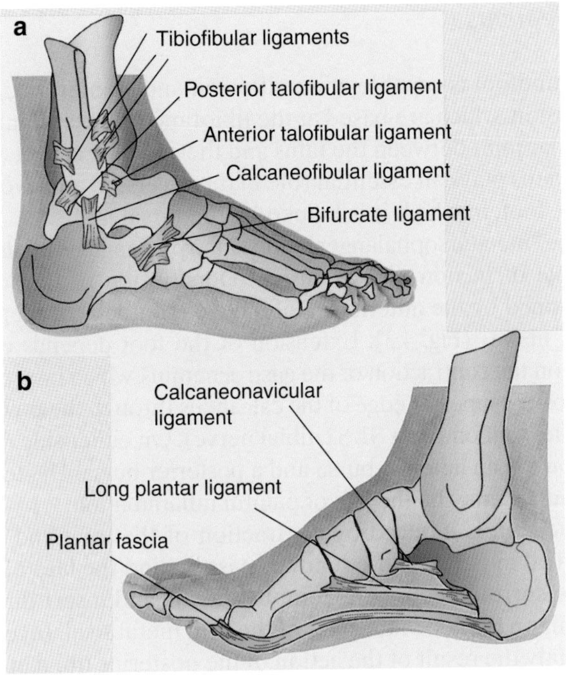

FIGURE 4.2 (**a**) Ligaments of the hindfoot (lateral aspect). (**b**) Antero-posterior arch and its ligaments

which may lead to inflammation at its posterior insertion – a common condition known as plantar fasciitis.

The loss of this anteroposterior arch results in so-called pes planus or flat foot. It may be accompanied by an outward deviation of the forefoot. It may be congenital, but is often found in patients with chronic arthritis as a result of laxity of the ligaments and collapse of the talonavicular joint.

There is also a transverse arch, which is more accentuated in the region of the tarsus and then continues more discreetly in the region of the metatarsophalangeal joints. Under normal conditions, the third and fourth metatarsophalangeal joints are not in contact with the ground. In patients with chronic arthritis such as rheumatoid arthritis, laxity of the ligaments may lead to collapse or even inversion of this arch, which results in painful calluses under the medial metatarsophalangeal joints.

Movements

The hindfoot is capable of dorsiflexion and plantar flexion or extension, which are based at the tibiotarsal (ankle) joint. The subtalar joint between the talus and the superior aspect of the calcaneus plays an essential role in the inversion and eversion of the foot, in which it is helped by the tarsal joints.

The metatarsophalangeal and interphalangeal joints are capable of flexion and extension. Dorsiflexion of the foot is performed by the anterior tibial muscle (root L4/L5, deep peroneal nerve) (Fig. 4.3). Extension of the foot depends essentially on the contraction of the gastrocnemius, which inserts into the posterosuperior edge of the calcaneus through the powerful Achilles tendon (root S1/S2, tibial nerve). On either side of this tendon are an anterior bursa and a posterior bursa. The tendon and bursae may be the site of painful inflammation.

Eversion is induced by contraction of the long and short peroneal muscles whose tendons pass behind the lateral malleolus, surrounded by a tendinous sheath, and insert through a common tendon at the base of the fifth metatarsal. Inversion is mainly the result of the action of the posterior tibial muscle, whose tendon passes behind the medial malleolus and inserts in the cuneiform bone. Fig. 11.12. shows the distribution of the cutaneous innervation of the foot.

The cutaneous and motor innervation of the toes is carried by nerves that are arranged between the metatarsals and metatarsophalangeals, where they may be subject to repeated traumatic lesions caused particularly by tight-fitting footwear. This causes Morton's meta - tarsalgia.

Radiological Anatomy

Anteroposterior and lateral radiographs of the ankle (Fig. 4.4.) give a clear view of the articular space, cortical edges and subchondral bone.

On the lateral, the insertion of the Achilles tendon is clearly visible and erosions and calcification may be evident.

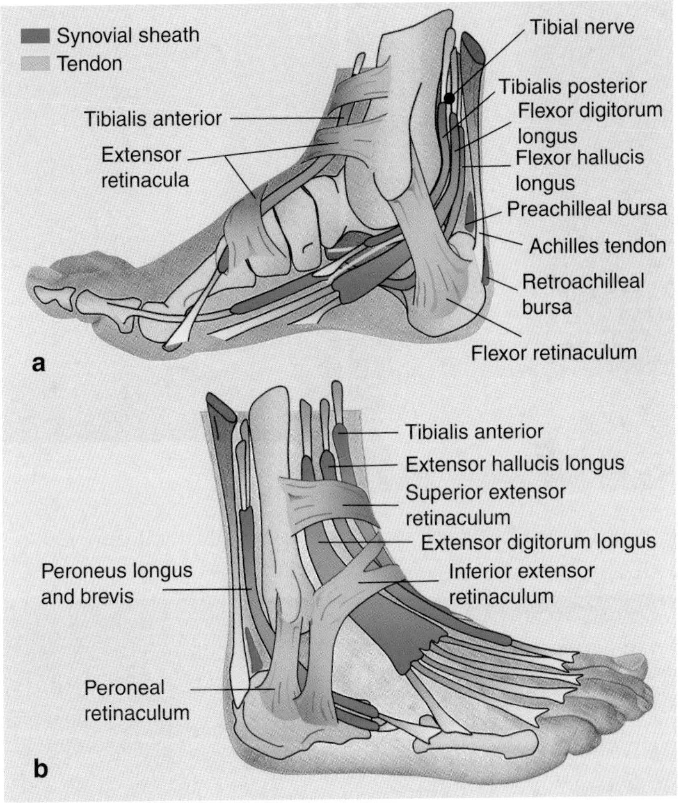

FIGURE 4.3 Tendons, synovial sheaths and bursae of the ankle and foot. (**a**) Medial aspect. (**b**) Lateral aspect

The subtalar and talonavicular joints may also be assessed from this plane.

An anteroposterior film of the foot gives a good view of the tarsometa - tarsal and metatarsophalangeal joints. Note the articular space and look for erosions or osteophytes. An oblique angle complements this study and gives a better view of the tarsal joints (Fig. 4.5). The interphalangeals are not easy to see in standard x-rays.

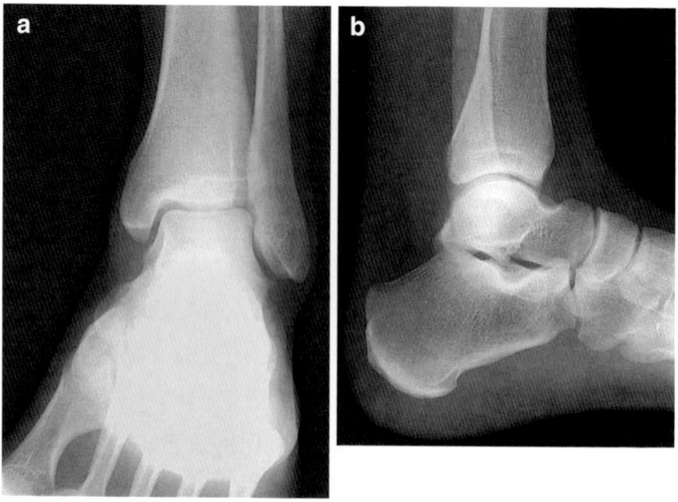

FIGURE 4.4 Ankle X-rays: antero-posterior and lateral view

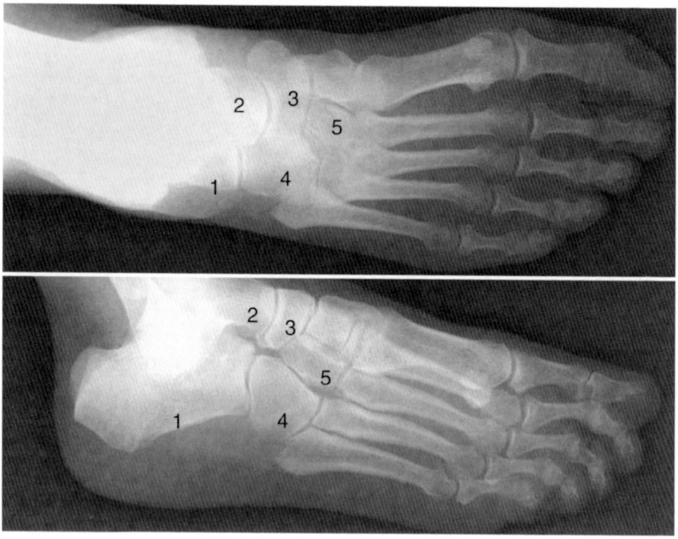

FIGURE 4.5 Foot X-rays: antero-posterior and oblique views. **1**. Calcaneus. **2**. Talus. **3**. Navicular **4**. Cuboid. **5**. Cuneiforms

Common Causes of Pain in the Foot and Ankle

Pain in the ankle and foot is frequently related to problems of footwear. Plantar fasciitis is commonly seen in middle-aged and elderly patients. In young people, traumatic lesions predominate. The most likely primary location of gout is in the first metatarsophalangeal joint (podagra), and is relatively common in middle-aged men (Table 4.1).

The joints in this area are often involved in different types of degenerative and inflammatory polyarthropathy. Note, however, that primary osteoarthritis only affects the tarsus and the first metatarsophalangeal joint with significant frequency. Its presence in other joints, including the tibiotarsal (ankle) joint, is rare and suggests osteoarthritis secondary, for example, to trauma, infection or other causes.

The Enquiry

The enquiry should focus on the aspects that are typical of each condition and on those that distinguish between them.

Where does it Hurt?

Table 4.1. shows the importance of this information. Generally speaking, pain in the ankle and foot is confined to one place and points to the injured structure.

Diffuse pain in the tarsus may be caused by local osteoarthritis or, more often, by changes in the structure of the foot or inappropriate footwear. Morton's metatar salgia may be described like this but, as a rule, is located further forward.

How did it Begin?

Acute onset of pain is to be expected in gout and sprains.

TABLE 4.1 The most common causes of pain in the ankle and foot.

Location	Nature of the lesion	Suggestive manifestations
Hindfoot	Plantar fasciitis	Pain in the plantar aspect of the hindfoot
		Exacerbated or triggered by load bearing
		Local tenderness
	Tendonitis of the Achilles tendon	Pain in the posterior aspect of the ankle
		Exacerbated by walking
		Local tenderness
	Sprain	Acute, post-traumatic onset
		Pain and functional disability
		Swelling and/or bruising
		Local tenderness
	Synovitis	Inflammatory pain
		Pain on palpation and motion
		Local warmth and swelling
Tarsus	Osteoarthritis	Mechanical pain
		Exacerbated by inversion and eversion
	Flat foot	Deep, ill-defined mechanical pain
		Flattening of the antero-posterior arch of the foot
Forefoot	Cavovarus foot	Deep, ill-defined mechanical pain
		Accentuation of the antero-posterior arch of the foot
	Morton's metatarsalgia	Mechanical, sometimes paresthetic pain
		Aggravated by tight-fitting shoes
		Pain on palpation between the metatarsals
	Hallux valgus	Mechanical pain over the big toe
		Valgus deformity of the first metatarsophalangeal joint
		Often associated with bursitis (bunions)
	Gout	Acute, recurring monoarthritis

TABLE 4.1 (continued)

Location	Nature of the lesion	Suggestive manifestations
		Predilection for the first metatarsophalangeal joint
	Metatarsophalangeal arthritis	Inflammatory pain Usual context of polyarthritis Local tenderness
	Dactylitis	Swelling and rubor of the whole toe ("sausage toe") Suggestive of psoriatic arthritis
	Toe deformities	Mechanical pain aggravated by footwear Visible deformity

Plantar fasciitis, Achilles tendonitis or bursitis, nonmicrocrystalline arthritis and dactylitis usually develop in days or weeks.

The pain in osteoarthritis, Morton's metatarsalgia, and foot or toe deformities usually develops over months or years before the patient seeks medical attention.

What is the Rhythm of the Pain?

Almost all the pain in this area is mechanical, either because of the degenerative nature of its source or because it is triggered by compression or distension of an inflamed structure, as in Achilles tendonitis and plantar fasciitis.

> Note that the pain caused by structural abnormalities of the feet is often accentuated at the first steps in the morning, gets better after a while and worsens again by the end of the day.

When the pain persists at rest, especially during the night, arthritis should be suspected.

Exacerbating Factors

Understandably, standing and walking are common exacerbating factors for pain in this area. Pain associated with the use of specific types of footwear (high heels, tight-fitting shoes) points to changes in structure or metatarsalgia. Arthritis of the metatarsophalangeals is also exacerbated in these circumstances.

Usual Footwear

Footwear plays a fundamental role in protecting the feet and unsuitable shoes are an extremely important factor in triggering acute pain and promoting chronic structural alterations. High heels overload the forefoot by transferring a lot of the weight to this area. Stiletto heels cause accentuated instability in the hindfoot and overload the local ligaments, frequently leading to repeated, chronic sprains. Tight-fitting, pointed shoes can obviously cause hallux valgus, facilitate the development of Morton's metatarsalgia and exacerbate pain related to deformities of the toes and arthritis of the forefoot.

Thin, hard soles cause repeated trauma of the soft structures and bones of the feet causing pain that may be relieved by wearing soft yet supportive, springy soles.

Repeated trauma of the Achilles tendon leading to tendonitis or bursitis may also be due to poor shoes.

Habits

Many occupations and leisure activities place intense, prolonged loads on the feet and demand superhuman resistance from them. This can be aggravated by irregular surfaces, tight, inflexible footwear and being overweight. Sometimes such simple facts need to be made clear to the patient.

Associated Manifestations

In general medicine, only rarely will ankle or foot swelling be related local inflammation. Venous insufficiency, heart, kidney or liver failure, and other causes of water retention are, by far, the commonest causes of lower limb edema. Typically, in these cases the edema tends to be bilateral and to predominate at the end of the day and after standing, and is improved in the morning or after resting with the legs raised. In arthritis of the ankle, the swelling is usually moderate and limited to the joint area. It is not relieved by rest. Gout causes accentuated local swelling with intense local heat and redness. In cases of concomitant pain and edema of the ankles or feet, it is essential to clarify the aspects.

The systematic enquiry will look mainly for articular manifestations in other places, especially when enthesopathy or arthritis is suspected as the cause of local pain (see manifestations of seronegative spondyloarthropathy). Associated diseases are also obviously important: heart failure in cases of edema, kidney stones in cases of gout, history of peptic ulcers, trauma, etc. Diabetes mellitus very often causes accentuated discomfort in the feet.

Note
In the presence of recurring enthesopathy of the feet in a young patient, seronegative spondyloarthropathy should always be considered.

The Local and Regional Examination

We suggest that you first conduct a general rheumatologic examination. An examination of the foot must include an assessment of the whole lower limb. If the patient complains about his or her ankle and foot, examination of this area should be more detailed. While paying special attention to the painful area, it is important to examine the patient's whole foot and his or her footwear.

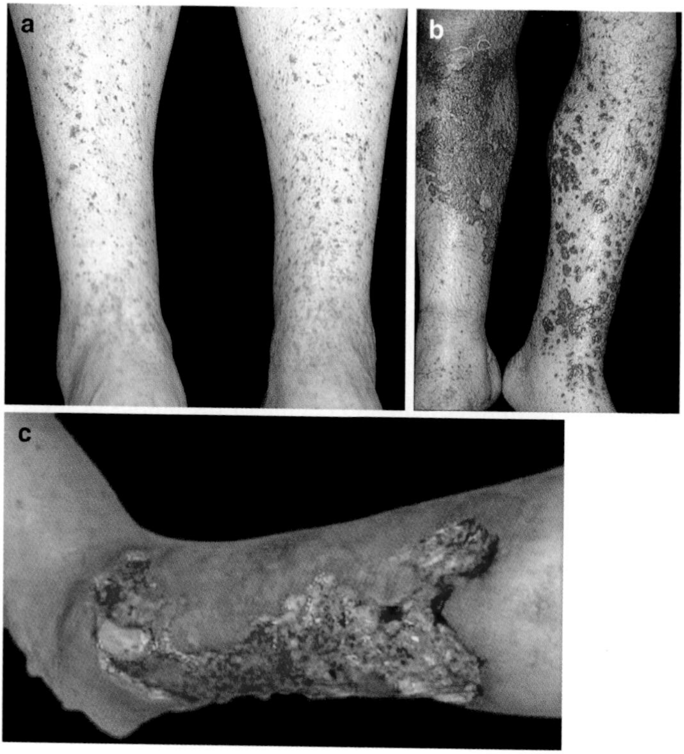

FIGURE 4.6 Skin lesions suggesting vasculitis. (**a**) Palpable purpura. (**b**) Hemorrhagic vesicles. (**c**) Ulceration

Inspection

Localized redness is almost exclusive to gout, dactylitis and infection. A diffuse purplish color or paleness, is a rare observation that suggests algodystrophy (see below) or Raynaud's phenomenon. The skin of the feet is a preferential location for lesions of vasculitis, which may consist of palpable purpura, bloody vesicles or even ulceration and gangrene (Fig. 4.6). Vasculitis is, however, very rare overall.

Ankle joint synovitis causes discreet swelling, which obliterates the normal depressions anterior and inferior to the medial and lateral malleoli.

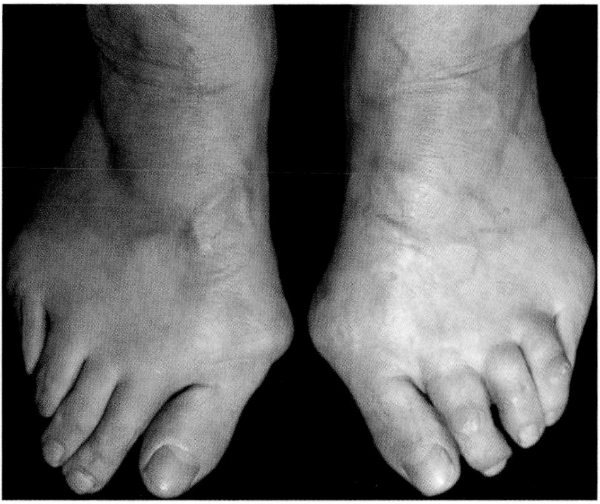

FIGURE 4.7 Hallux valgus in a patient with rheumatoid arthritis. Note also the loss of the transverse arch of the forefoot

Dystrophy of the toenails may be due to mycosis or psoriasis.

Note the alignment of the hallux: accentuated lateral deviation (hallux valgus) is a common cause of local pain (Fig. 4.7). It is often accompanied by an inflammatory reaction of the bursa that covers the medial face of the first metatarsophalangeal joint: the associated bursitis is commonly known as a bunion. Assess the other toes for deformities that may explain pain (Fig. 4.8). Examine the soles of the feet, looking for calluses. They are important especially if they are not in the usual places (under the calcaneus, the first or fifth metatarsophalangeal joints).

Outside these locations, calluses suggest deformity of the foot or inadequate footwear. Flatness or inversion of the transverse arch of the forefoot may be evaluated with the patient lying on his back and is almost always associated with calluses under the third and/or fourth metatarsophalangeal joints (Fig. 4.7).

Alterations in the structure or dynamics of the foot are easier to assess when the patient is standing:

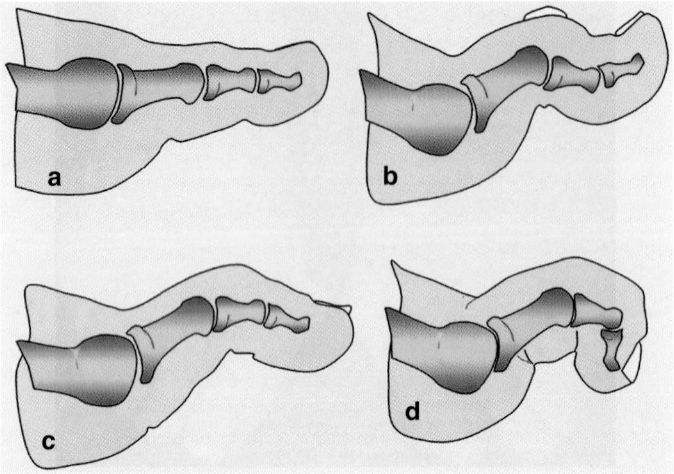

FIGURE 4.8 Deformities of the toes. (**a**) Normal. (**b**) Hammer. (**c**) Mallet toe. (**d**) Claw toe

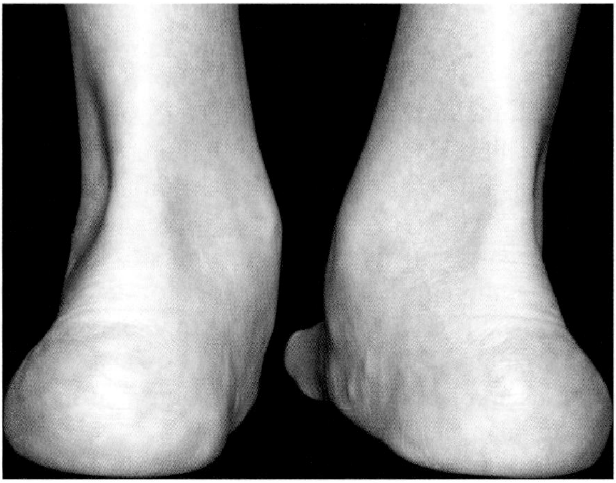

FIGURE 4.9 Calcaneo valgus in a patient with rheumatoid arthritis.

- Examine the position of the axis of the heel in relation to the lower leg. External deviation (calcaneus valgus) is very common, especially in patients with chronic arthritis (Fig. 4.9.);

- Under normal conditions, the medial edge of the foot is arched so there is a space between it and the ground when the patient is standing. Absence or reduction of this distance means flat foot. An exaggerated longitudinal arch is typical of cavovarus foot.

Palpation

Explore the articular space on the anterior aspect of the tibiotarsal joint. The edges of the joint curve backwards, making them hard to palpate. In cases of synovitis this space is full with an elastic and tender tissue. Swelling and pain around the malleoluses are also common. Firm palpation of inflammatory swelling does not leave any "pitting," unlike vascular edema.

In the case of hindfoot pain, carefully palpate the inferior insertion of the Achilles tendon and adjoining structures. In tendonitis or bursitis, palpation is painful, and is sometimes accompanied by local edema. In plantar fasciitis there is pain on deep palpation at its posterior insertion in the calcaneus (Fig. 4.10).

If these areas are painless, palpate along the posterior face of the internal and external malleoli looking for tenosynovitis of the posterior tibial and peroneal muscles, respectively. The tibial nerve passes behind the medial malleolus. Rarely, its compression here can cause tarsal tunnel syndrome, with paresthetic pain in the sole of the foot. This is the place for Tinel's test.

Perform the metatarsal "squeeze"test, applying pressure across the metatarsophalangeal joints transversely. This maneuver is painful in local synovitis, metatarsalgia, hallux valgus and bunions. If there is pain, you should then focus the palpation on each individual MTP joint, putting your thumb on its dorsal face and your index finger on the plantar face (Fig. 4.11a). Look for swelling, deformity and pain.

In Morton's metatarsalgia, transverse compression of the foot causes pain between two adjacent metatarsals. Deep

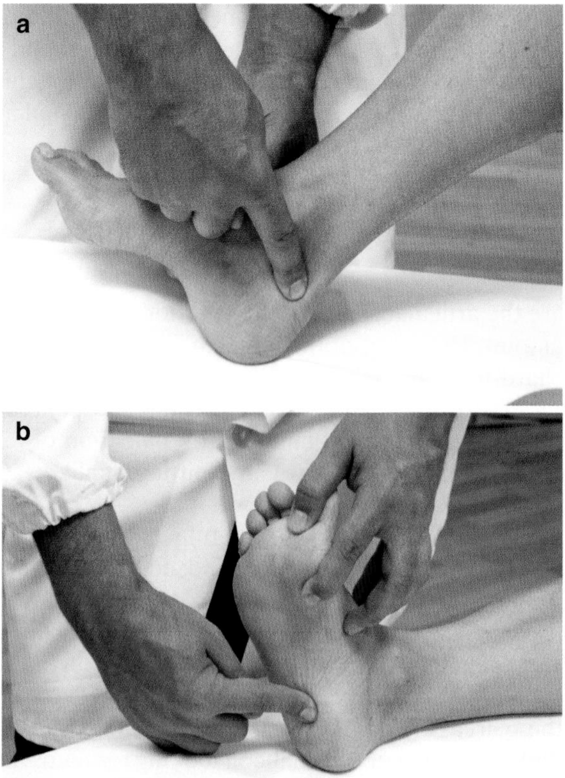

FIGURE 4.10 (**a**) Palpation of the Achilles tendon and preachillean bursa. (**b**) Palpation of the posterior insertion of plantar fascia

palpation along the spaces between the metatarsals is painful, and may be accompanied by paresthesia of the corresponding toes (Fig. 4.11b).

The first metatarsophalangeal is often the site of osteoarthritis, generally associated with hallux valgus. The bursa that covers it is often inflamed and painful. It is also a common site for gouty tophi.

The interphalangeal joints of the feet are difficult to examine, but may be painful in cases of arthritis or repeated trauma.

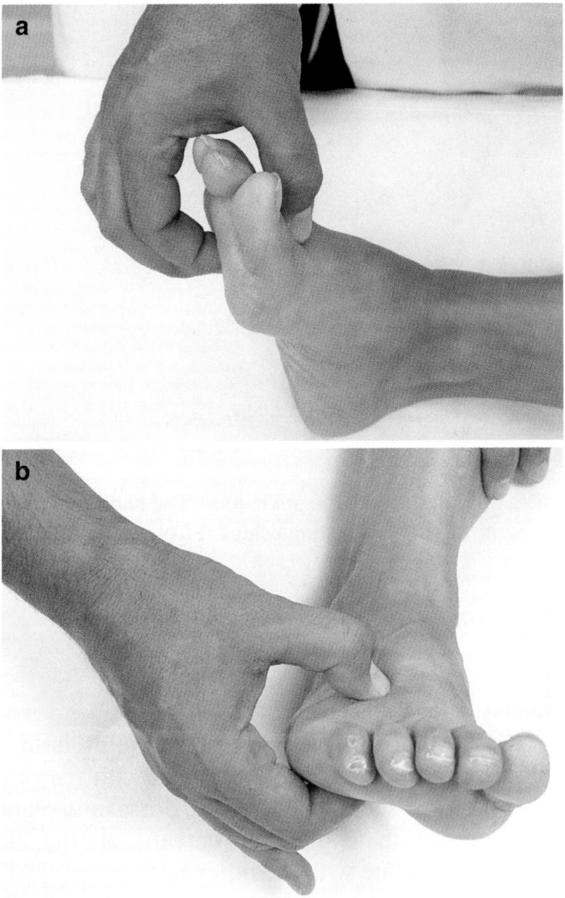

FIGURE 4.11 (**a**) Individual palpation of metatarsophalangeal joints. (**b**) Palpation of intermetatarsal spaces - painful in Morton's metatarsalgia

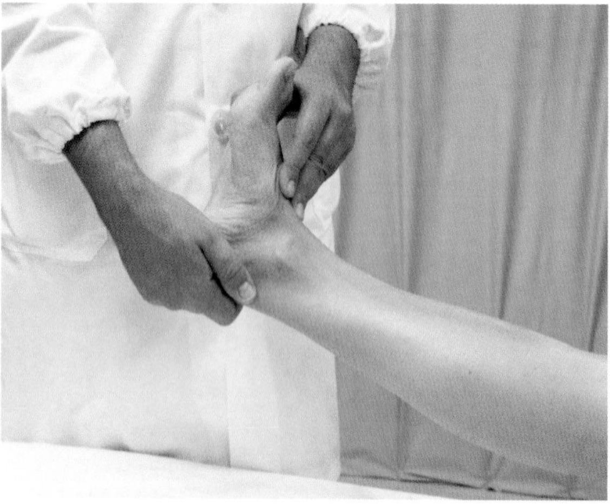

FIGURE 4.12 Mobilization of the ankle joint. The hand that grasps the heel moves the ankle joint, distinguishing it from that of the midfoot

Mobilization

1. Mobility of the ankle joint

To assess the mobility of the tibiotarsal joint, hold the heel firmly with one hand and the tibia with the other, keeping the knee semi-flexed. Induce dorsal and plantar flexion and evaluate the movements of the heel (Fig. 4.12).[1] Compare with the other side.

Normal dorsiflexion goes up to 15–25° and extension from 40 to 50°: limited mobility indicates articular and not periarticular abnormality.

[1]The tarsus also has flexion and extension movements. Immobilizing the heel enables us to isolate the movements of the tibiotarsal joint and evaluate them separately.

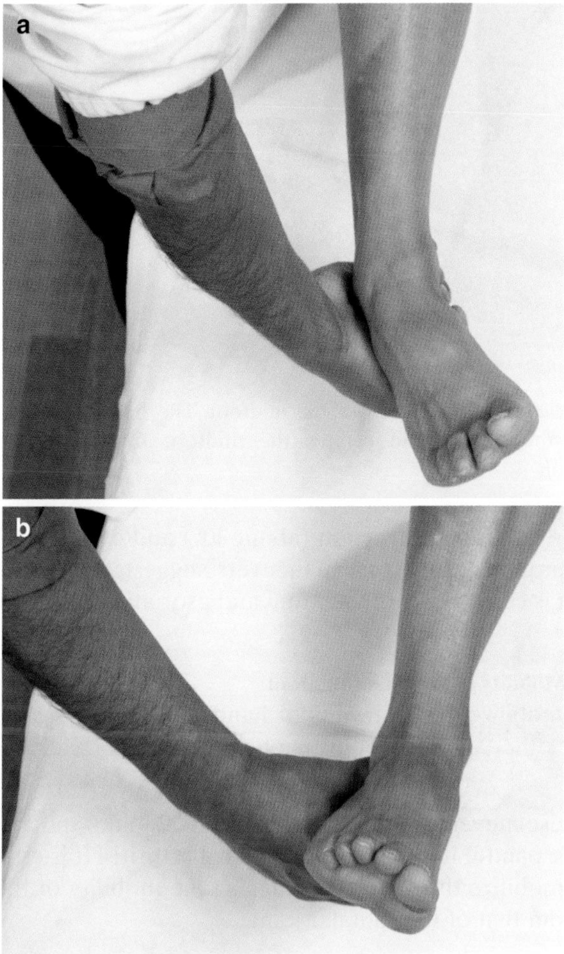

FIGURE 4.13 Mobilization of the subtalar joint. Hold firmly the heel and induce movements of inversion (**a**) and eversion (**b**)

2. Mobility of the subtalar joint
Firmly holding the heel, induce inversion and eversion (Fig. 4.13). Compare with the other side.

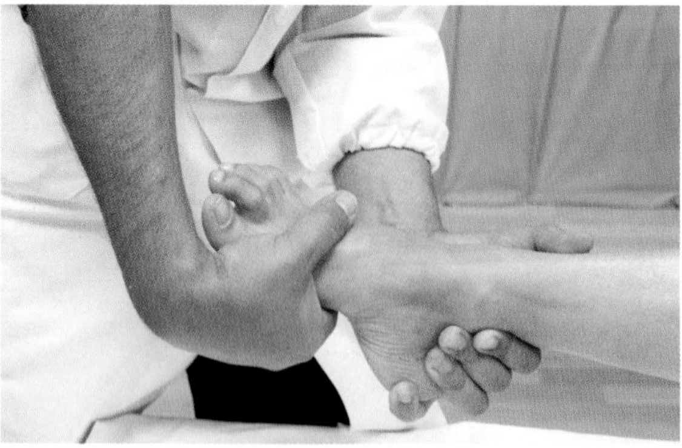

FIGURE 4.14 Mobilization of the midfoot. The heel is immobilized while the other hand rotates the midfoot into inversion and eversion

A reduction in inversion (about 40°) and eversion (about 15°), or pain during these maneuvers, suggests local synovitis, which is common in rheumatoid and psoriatic arthritis.

3. Mobility of the tarsus/midfoot
Immobilize the heel with one hand. Hold the tarsus with the other and induce inversion and eversion (Fig. 4.14).

These movements depend on the tarsal joints and are limited or painful in the presence of local arthritis. It is essential to immobilize the heel to distinguish the mobility of the tarsus from that of the subtalar joint.

4. Global active motion of the foot and ankle
Now ask the patient to turn his feet up and then down as far possible. Compare the two sides.

A reduction in these movements can be explained by alterations already found in the ankle or tarsus. If the limitation is much more than expected, we should consider the possibility of retraction of the Achilles tendon or of the dorsiflexors.

The Neurological Examination

Pain in the foot may be caused by nerve root compression (sciatica). Lesions due to peripheral neuropathy, which are common in diabetes, for example, can also cause local pain, which is usually paraesthetic and diffuse. Both neuropathies and sciatica can be accompanied by reduced or absent Achilles reflexes. When the alteration is unilateral, its pathological significance is more certain, reflecting a root or peripheral nerve lesion. In peripheral neuropathies, the alteration is usually bilateral. We should, however, bear in mind that the Achilles reflexes of many elderly patients are almost or completely unreactive, even in the absence of disease.

If you suspect a neurogenic lesion, test the sensitivity to pain of the feet and lower legs: a symmetrical, sock-shaped distribution of loss is typical of peripheral neuropathy. Localized loss affecting a dermatome may be due to nerve root or peripheral nerve lesion, depending on the affected area (Fig. 11.12).

It is easier to assess muscle strength with the patient standing. Ask him to take a few steps on tiptoe (gastrocnemius, S1/S2) or on his heels (anterior tibial, L4/L5).

Please note: It can be useful to look at the patient's shoes, provided that they are not new.

Asymmetrical wear of the heel indicates a dynamic imbalance. Deformation of a shoe can be a clear indication of a varus or valgus deviation of the hindfoot, hallux valgus, deformed toes or a collapsed transverse arch, for example.

Typical Cases

4.A. Heel Pain (I)

Rosário Domingos, a normally healthy 52-year old cook, went to her doctor because of pain in her left foot that was making it difficult to work. The progressive onset of the pain, which was mainly located in the heel, had begun two months before, increasing in intensity until she could not stand on it for any length of time. It was particularly intense when she took the first steps in the morning and went away soon after. It was exacerbated by prolonged standing. She had not noticed any relationship with footwear. She was much better wearing trainers.

She denied any other important manifestations and had had no treatment.

On clinical examination, we found her to be obese, with no other relevant alterations.

The foot, examined with the patient lying down and standing, had no apparent deformities and the arches were normal. There were accentuated calluses on the inferior face of both heels. Articular mobility was normal and painless.

Plantar Fasciitis

Main Points

Consists of the inflammation of the posterior insertion of the plantar fascia in the calcaneal tuberosity, with or without associated bursitis.

It is common in middle-aged men and women.

Being overweight, having flat feet, prolonged standing and walking and irregular surfaces are risk factors.

It may occasionally be a manifestation of seronegative spondyloarthropathy.

It is reflected by plantar pain in the hindfoot, aggravated by weightbearing.

The local examination makes the diagnosis.

In the absence of other manifestations, there is no place for plain films. Ultrasound and MRI scans may help with a doubtful diagnosis.

Treatment consists of reducing compression and local trauma through rest, weight loss and special insoles (Fig. 4.15). Suggest soft yet firm, supportive, properly shaped footwear.

In persistent situations, a local injection may be necessary.

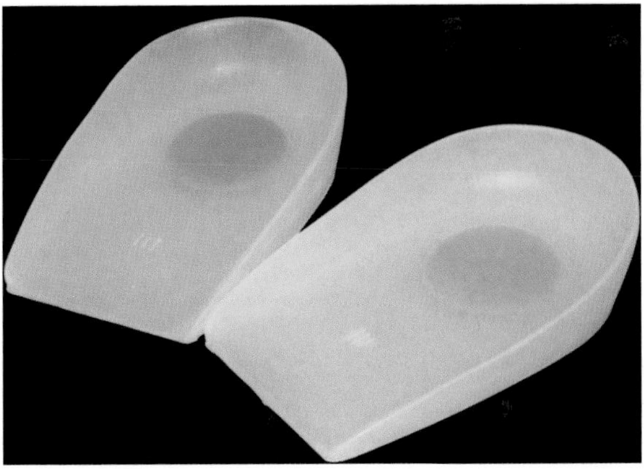

FIGURE 4.15 Insoles used in the treatment of plantar fasciitis – the area corresponding to the posterior insertion of the fascia (blue) is softer, to avoid compressing the painful structure

Heel spur

We mention this merely to devalue it. This is a bony growth that is often seen in radiographs at the point of plantar fascia insertion in the calcaneus (Fig. 4.16).

Although many doctors tend to consider this anomaly to be a source of pain or plantar fasciitis, in practical terms it is unrelated to the symptoms. The patient has plantar fasciitis if we find the above symptoms, even if the x-ray is normal. The patient does not have plantar fasciitis if the clinical examination does not indicate it, even if s/he has a spur. We therefore suggest that you not attach any significance to this radiographic finding.

Did we know enough for a diagnosis?
What else would you have done?

Palpation of the inferior face of the heel was diffusely painful, but triggered intense pain at the lower anterior edge of the calcaneus. The inferior insertion of the Achilles tendon was normal on inspection and palpation.

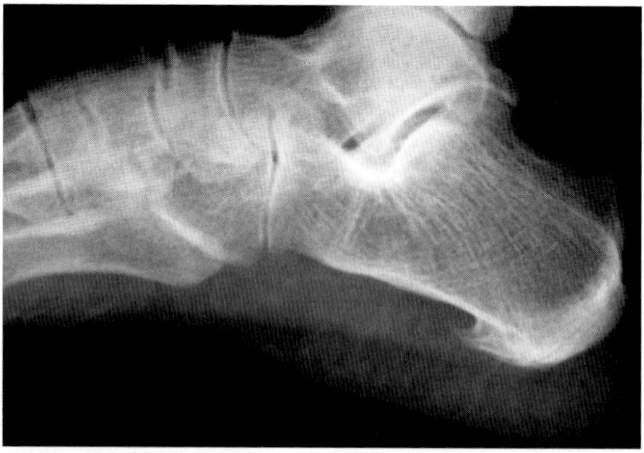

FIGURE 4.16 Calcaneal spur. It is a common radiological image with no clinical relevance

What is your diagnosis?

What advice would you give the patient?

We concluded that the patient had plantar fasciitis. We explained the situation to her and stressed the relationship between her complaint and being overweight and prolonged standing and walking. Such conditions can cause pain even in the absence of fasciitis! We prescribed a pair of doughnut-shaped insoles to take the load off the insertion of the fascia. We recommended partial rest and loss of weight.

We suggested that she wear well-cushioned shoes with thick, flexible rubber soles providing support for the longitudinal arch (good-quality trainers/sneakers would be a good choice). We arranged to see the patient again if her condition did not improve and prepared her for the possibility of a local corticosteroid injection.

Typical Cases

4.B. Heel Pain (II)

David Paiva, a 21-year old student, came to us because of pain in the posterior face of his right heel, which had begun about three months before and had become progressively worse. The pain was more intense when he walked, and especially while playing football or going downstairs. He had nocturnal discomfort and it was much worse in the morning. He described swelling of the Achilles tendon/posterior aspect of heel.

Our systematic enquiry revealed that he had also been suffering back pain for two or three years, especially after long periods of immobility at his desk. He had occasional morning pain. He denied any other articular or extra-articular manifestations except for asthmatic bronchitis that he had had for a long time and was well controlled.

The clinical examination of his feet suggested slight swelling of the inferior insertion of the right Achilles tendon, with marked tenderness on local palpation. Mobilization caused pain on forced dorsiflexion of the right ankle joint, with painful limitation of the range of movement.

Give a brief description of the relevant problems.[2]
What is your diagnosis?
What treatment would you suggest?

We concluded that David had tendonitis of the Achilles tendon with associated bursitis.

We suggested that he wore shoes with a higher heel for some time to relax the tendon somewhat. We advised him to stop playing football and other strenuous exercise for a while and prescribed a topical antiinflammatory.

We stressed the importance in the future of warming-up exercises and stretching the tendons before any more strenuous exercise.

We arranged to see him again 3 weeks later.

---

[2] Achilles tendonitis in a young man with a history of back pain.

Achilles Tendonitis/Bursitis

Main Points

This is the inflammation of the inferior insertion of the Achilles tendon and/or of the pre- and retro-Achilles bursae. It is most common in young males.

It causes local pain that is exacerbated by walking, especially going downstairs, as this involves greater distension of the tendon.

Strenuous sports, inappropriate footwear and seronegative spondyloarthropathy are important risk factors.

Pain on local palpation, exacerbated by forced dorsiflexion, confirms the diagnosis. There may be local swelling.

Repeated episodes weaken the tendon and may lead to partial or total rupture.

Ultrasound and MRI scans are useful in assessing the tendon's condition, especially in chronic inflammation or suspected rupture.

The initial treatment involves resting the tendon with raised heels, topical anti-inflammatories and partial physical rest.

Stubborn cases may benefit from oral NSAIDs or demand the use of physical agents, stretching exercises or a splint in physiotherapy.

Local steroid injections are associated with increased risk of tendon rupture and should only be avoided.

Typical Cases

4.C. Pain In The Forefoot (I)

It was the third time that it had happened: intense pain over the first metatarsophalangeal joint that appeared at night after going to bed quite well. The joint swelled and went red and the slightest touch caused excruciating pain. The first two episodes, which had occurred the year before, had been on the other foot and responded in about 4 days to NSAIDs prescribed at emergency.

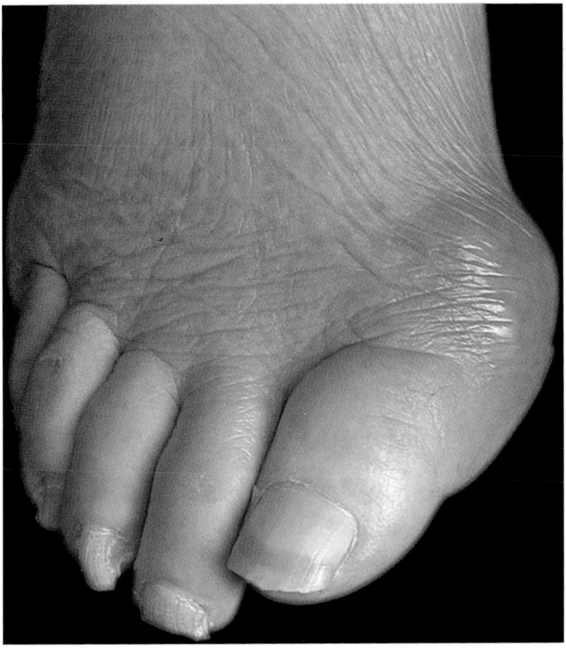

FIGURE 4.17 Clinical case "Pain in the forefoot (I)." Notice the swelling and redness of the first metarso-phalangeal joint

Manuel, a 45-year old farmer, wondered what the problem was and how it would develop.

He denied any similar episodes in other joints. He had a history of kidney stones (a single episode 3 years before) and well controlled hypertension. He confessed that he normally ate rather too much and often drank alcohol.

His late father had had severe articular problems similar to his, but they also affected other joints.

There were no other significant abnormalities in our clinical examination. The examination of the foot confirmed monoarthritis of the first right MTP, which was frankly swollen, hot and painful (Fig. 4.17). There did not seem to be any articular effusion, so we did not conduct an arthrocentesis.

Were we missing anything?[3]
What do you think are the probable diagnoses?
On what basis?
Would you request any tests?
How would you treat this situation?

We reached a diagnosis of **acute gouty arthritis,** and prescribed a full dose of anti-inflammatories to be taken regularly until the pain ceased.

We requested routine lab tests, including serum urate level, serum lipids, liver enzymes, creatinine and 24-hour uricosuria. The patient was instructed to have these tests a few weeks after the end of this crisis.

He came to clinic again 4 weeks later as agreed. The flare-up had responded to the medication with no recurrences. The lab tests showed elevated uricemia at 9.4 mg/dl, with hypertriglyceridemia and elevated γ-GT. The uricosuria was normal.

This confirmed our suspected diagnosis.[4] We discussed the highly probable relationship of the disease with his eating and drinking habits, stressing the need to moderate his protein intake and give up alcohol. Allopurinol would be started in the future if these measures proved insufficient. The patient promised to comply…

Gouty Arthritis
Main Points
This is the inflammation of a joint in reaction to deposition of monosodium urate crystals. It occurs most commonly in middle-aged men.

---

[3] Very good! We have a young man with Achilles tendonitis with no apparent cause. But he has a suspicious backache. In fact, although we might think that his back pain was postural, from an incorrect position while sitting, it is inflammatory: after rest and sometimes in the morning. We had to consider the possibility of seronegative spondyloarthropathy, and especially ankylosing spondylitis, of which the tendonitis would another sign (enthesopathy). And this was, indeed, the case with our patient.

[4] A positive diagnosis had to wait for a sample of synovial fluid showing the presence of uric acid crystals.

It is rare in post-menopausal women and exceptional in young women.

It usually starts with episodes of acute, recurring monoarthritis, with clear signs of inflammation, separated by asymptomatic intervals.

The first MTP is the site of the first episode in about 50% of cases (podagra). The tarsus is also often affected. With time it tends to involve more proximal joints and even the upper limb.

The diagnosis is essentially clinical and is reinforced by findings of hyperuricemia.

The final diagnosis is established by demonstration of monosodium urate crystals in the synovial fluid.

A more detailed clinical description of gout and its treatment is given in Chap. 18.

Typical Cases

4.D. Pain In The Forefoot (II)

"My feet are killing me," answered the patient when I asked her why she had come to see us. She described "excruciating" pain in both feet that had become worse over several years. It had recently become unbearable in her right foot, preventing her from working in her boutique. The longstanding pain was typically mechanical and was located in the first MTP. It was particularly bad in the morning when she put her shoes on and got worse again at the end of the day. It was distinctly less severe during the weekends, when she wore her favorite slippers.

Recently the pain in her right foot had changed significantly. It was more intense and affected the whole forefoot. Sometimes, she even had what felt like an electric shock and had to take off her shoes in the middle of the shop! The pain was less intense at night, though it sometimes woke her up.

She denied any other relevant symptoms.

Think about the possible diagnoses at this stage.
Plan the clinical examination.

In the clinical examination, I noted her elegant, high-heeled shoes with thin soles and pointed toes. The hallux deviated considerably in both feet, pushing against the second toe. The little toe was bent inwards. On the medial aspect of the right first MTP there was a slightly reddish swelling that fluctuated on palpation. Mobilization of the hallux was painful, with crepitus that was more accentuated on the left.

Examination of the left tarsus revealed no alterations. Deep palpation between the third and fourth right metatarsals, however, caused intense pain at a well defined point, reproducing the characteristics of the recent spontaneous pain.

Hallux Valgus

Main Points

This is a very common condition in middle-aged and elderly women.

It consists of the inward deviation of the first metatarsophalangeal joint.

It is associated with a congenital predisposition, but is further exacerbated by ill-fitting shoes.

Traumatic bursitis on the medial face of the joint ("bunions") is a common complication.

It causes local pain, which is exacerbated by walking and ill-fitting shoes and may radiate to neighboring areas.

In an anteroposterior radiograph of the foot, the diagnosis is confirmed if the angle between the first metatarsal and the big toe is larger than 10~15°.

Treatment involves wearing well-fitted, supportive shoes without pointed toes and having restraining features to prevent the toes sliding forward, reducing the load on them. Persistent bursitis may respond to a local injection.

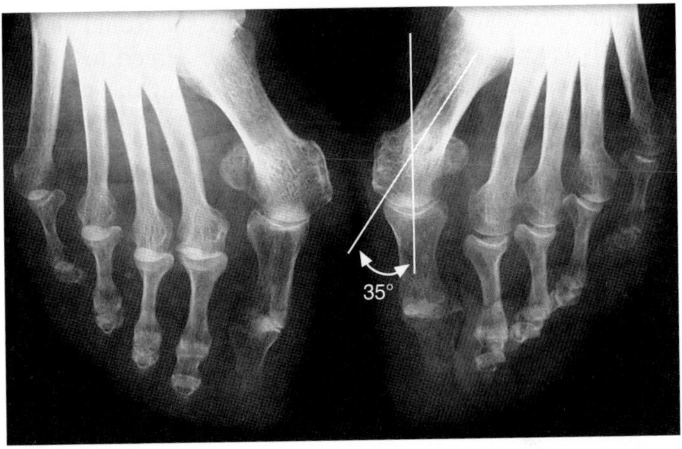

FIGURE 4.18 Clinical case "Pain in the forefoot (II)." Note the deviation of the first metatarsal bone, bilaterally. The 1st MTP joint presents features of osteoarthritis. The exostosis of the medial aspect of first metatarsal bone testifies the intensity and duration of local compression by shoes

Left untreated hallux valgus will almost always leads to osteoarthritis of the first MTP, with mechanical pain that no longer responds to simple measures.

Surgical correction, which is reserved for stubborn, incapacitating cases, usually has good results.

What are the probable diagnoses at this stage?

What treatment would you recommend?

We explained the cause of her suffering to the patient: bilateral hallux valgus, with bursitis, probable osteoarthritis and Morton's metatarsalgia on the right. Indeed, the plain film that she had with her showed osteoarthritis the hallux valgus (Fig. 4.18).

We stressed the role that her choice of footwear had played and encouraged her to change to comfortable shoes with flexible soles, low heels, malleable leather and wide at the front. The patient balked at this. We explained that if she continued to wear the same kind of shoes, she would almost certainly have continuing severe pain. She agreed to a local injection of anesthetic and a corticosteroid at the point of maximum pain between the metatarsals, followed by bed rest for 24 hours.

She came back a few months later and said that the pain was much better with the suggested changes. The paraesthetic pain in her right foot persisted, however. Our local examination was the same. We requested an ultrasound of the foot, which confirmed Morton's neurinoma. The patient opted for surgery.

Morton's Metatarsalgia

Main Points

This condition is relatively common in middle-aged and elderly women.

It is caused by the compression of the interdigital nerves of the foot, usually between the third and fourth metatarsals. In some patients there is a fibrous nodule (Morton's neuroma), which is visible on ultrasound.

This condition is responsible for intense pain in the forefoot, exacerbated by standing and ill-fitting shoes. It is sometimes dysesthetic.

Firm palpation between the metatarsals reproduces the spontaneous pain. Rarely, there may be an alteration in sensitivity to pain in the corresponding toes.

Ultrasound scan can be necessary to clarify a doubtful case or to support decisions regarding surgery. Initial treatment is conservative and based on more appropriate footwear and achieving an ideal weight. It stubborn cases, surgery may be considered.

Typical Cases

4.E. Heel Pain (III)

It was not really pain that she felt, but rather an ache of the right ankle, with a frequent "wobbly" feeling. The

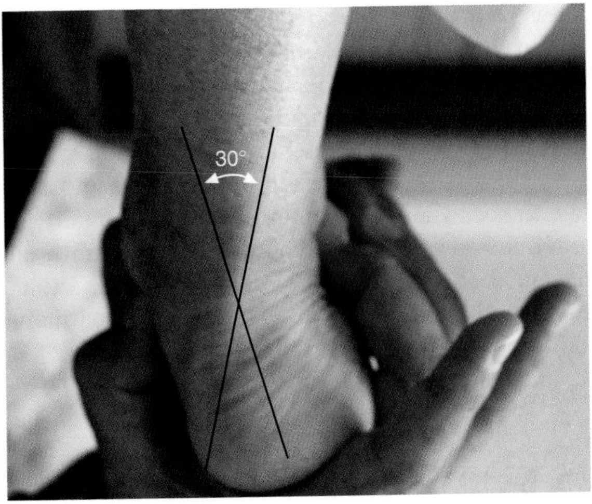

FIGURE 4.19 Clinical case "Hell pain (III)." Forced eversion of the heel

problems predominated at the end of a whole day on her feet, said this 47-year old teacher. She complained of occasional swelling in the painful ankle, mainly in the evening, which eased after a few days of partial rest. She normally wore flat shoes, not because she liked them, but because she could not tolerate high heels.

She denied any associated manifestations. Her past clinical history was not significant. When we persisted, she remembered a sprain in that foot when she was at school. She had had to rest for a few days, but had recovered fully.

Examination of the lower limbs showed the alignment to be normal. Mobility of the feet and ankles was normal. Eversion of the right foot was much more accentuated than the left. Firmly holding her heel with our fingers under the malleoluses, we found that forced eversion caused pain under the internal malleolus (Fig. 4.19). There were no other abnormalities.

What is your diagnosis?

Would it be worth requesting any diagnostic tests?

What treatment would you suggest?

We explained to the patient that she very likely had a chronic rupture of the ligaments in the medial side of the ankle. We suggested she wore supportive shoes and an elastic bandage to keep the heel in neutral position.

The requested ultrasound scan confirmed a rupture of the tibiocalcaneal and posterior tibiotalar ligament. The patient clearly gained relief with the suggested treatment and decided to postpone consideration of surgery.

Ankle Sprain And Chronic Instability

Main Points

An acute ankle sprain consists of the total or partial rupture of the articular ligaments, due to excessive force in inversion or, more rarely, eversion.

It causes acute, incapacitating pain, with subsequent swelling and/or bruising.

Mild cases can be treated with rest, icepacks, compression and elevation of the limb, with a slow return to normal activities.

Patients who cannot bear weight or present accentuated swelling, bruising or signs of instability should be referred urgently to an orthopedic surgeon.

Persistence of an untreated rupture results in chronic articular instability, with mechanical pain and recurrent flares. The ankle joint may develop osteoarthritis.

Clinical examination reveals lateral or anteroposterior instability (drawer sign).

Initial treatment of chronic instability is conservative, involving stable, well-cushioned shoes and an elastic bandage.

Stabilizing surgery may be necessary.

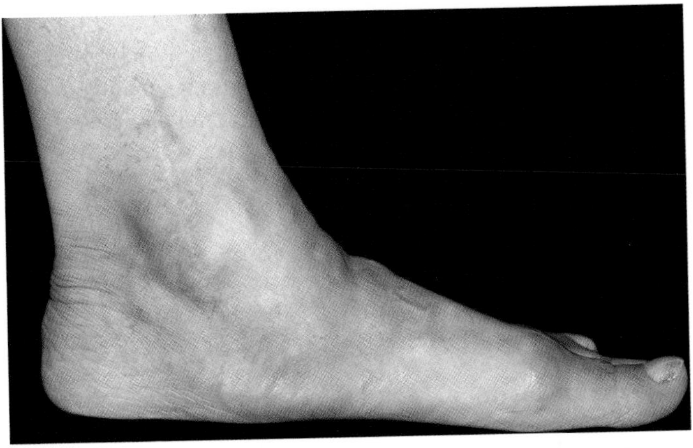

FIGURE 4.20 Clinical case "Diffuse mechanical pain." Note the loss of the antero-posterior arch of the foot, with medial and plantar displacement of the talus and navicular bones

Typical Cases

4.F. Diffuse Mecanical Pain

Dr. Manuela Fragoso, a 38-year old gastroenterologist, came to us because of pain in both feet that was making her medical work difficult. She had had the pain for a long time, since adolescence, but it had got progressively worse. It usually appeared on days when she stood or walked a lot and she sometimes had to sit down and massage her feet. The pain was diffuse but particularly affected the tarsus. She had begun to wear orthopedic sandals at work but without much relief. She had suffered a fracture of the right medial malleolus when she was 24.

Examination of the fee, with the patient lying on her back, showed no alterations other than enlargement of the forefeet and discreet, bilateral calluses under the third MTP. Palpation of the soles caused discreet discomfort along the medial edge. The anterior ends of the talus and the navicular bone were palpable on the medial edge of the foot. Articular mobility was normal and painless. Examination with the patient standing revealed flat feet, with almost all the foot in contact with the floor (Fig. 4.20). The curvature reappeared when the patient stood on tiptoe, showing flexibility of the tarsal joints.

Flat Feet And Cavovarus Foot

Main Points

These are deformities of the feet with a reduction (flat foot) or heightened (cavovarus foot) arch of the foot.

Most cases are asymptomatic, but they are a common cause of pain in young adults.

Flat foot usually also involves loss of the transversal arch of the forefoot, with the formation of painful calluses.

Cavovarus foot is often associated with claw or hammer toe and with local trauma and pain.

Both may be congenital or acquired.

The diagnosis is clinical but can be confirmed by podoscopy or a lateral weight-bearing radiograph, for an exact measurement of the angle of the internal arch (Fig. 4.21).

The treatment is essentially conservative, using insoles and/or well-shaped, flexible footwear to achieve better weight distribution.

If the problems persist, consider referring the patient to a podiatrist for custom-made insoles.

Surgery is reserved for extreme, incapacitating cases that do not respond to conservative measures.

What would you recommend to this patient?

The orthopedic sandals that she wore were well-shaped but made of hard, inflexible material.

We suggested softer, more malleable footwear, with insoles to reinforce the longitudinal arch of her feet, or comfortable,

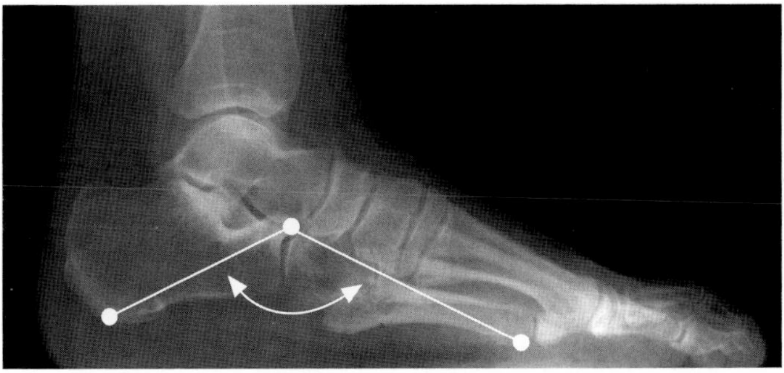

FIGURE 4.21 Pes planus and pes cavus. Radiological diagnosis based on weight-bearing radiographs: References: lowest point of the calcaneus; lowest point of the talus and lowest point of the head of the 1st metatarsal bone. Normal: 115 ~ 125°. (Courtesy: Prof. Caseiro Alves.)

loose trainers/sneakers, possibly one size larger than normal. She would certainly have to continue alternating rest and standing. The most drastic solution involved surgical correction, which we would reassess on the basis of the results achieved with these measures.

Special Situations

Rheumatoid Foot

The foot is a particularly important site of pain and disability in rheumatoid arthritis patients. The metatarsophalangeal joints are among those affected early, frequently and severely in this disease. This involvement is reflected by localized inflammatory pain, which may be a presenting feature or appear subsequently in the context of polyarthritis. Transverse squeezing of the forefeet and individual palpation of these joints causes pain and may reveal synovial inflammation. MTP joints are often the first site of bone erosions on x-rays, developing into progressive joint destruction (Fig. 4.22).

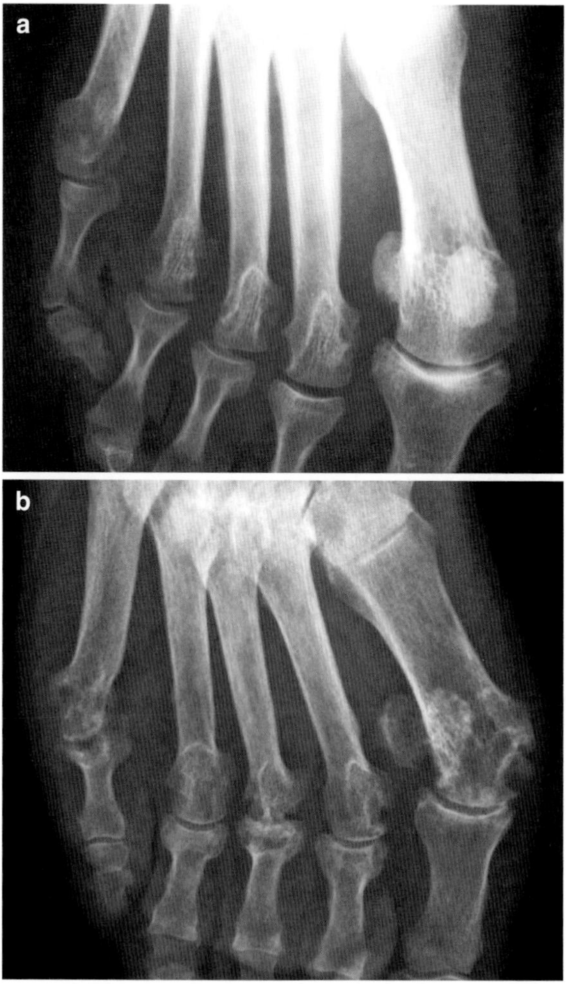

FIGURE 4.22 Radiographs of the feet in rheumatoid arthritis. (**a**) Patient with symptoms for eight months. Notice the erosions in all MTP joints. (**b**) Patient with disease for 5 years. Profound disorganization of the joints

The ankle and subtalar joints are also commonly affected. The subtalar joints are particularly susceptible to early, irreversible destruction of the cartilage and bone, which may cause considerable pain and disability.

In untreated rheumatoid arthritis the feet tend to acquire a variety of deformities which are, in themselves, causes of progressive, incapacitating pain even if the inflammatory process is controlled after they are established. The most common of these deformities are calcaneus valgus (Fig. 4.23a), "triangular"forefoot with hallux valgus and crossed toes (Fig. 4.23b) and secondary flat foot, with collapsed talonavicular joint and painful calluses under the third and fourth MTPs (Fig. 4.24).

Given the impact of walking on quality of life, the rheumatoid patient's feet warrant special care, based first and foremost on early, aggressive treatment of the disease, with cautious use of local injections, if necessary. Once deformities are established, we are faced with a difficult, highly incapacitating problem requiring a multidisciplinary approach, frequently with disappointing results.

Diabetic Foot

The feet of diabetic patients require very special care. Alterations caused by macro-and microvasculature changes expose patients to painful trophic skin alterations with a high risk of infection.

Polyneuropathy, which is common in these patients, may result in symptoms suggesting rheumatic disease, with diffuse pain and paresthesia. Impairment of deep sensitivity leads to disturbances of articular stability and muscle imbalance with pain and a predisposition to deformity and secondary osteoarthritis. In later stages, with accentuated loss of deep sensitivity, Charcot's arthropathy may set in, heralded in the early stages by signs of acute inflammation reminiscent of gout but with a notable absence of pain. Over time, this condition leads to total malposition of the joint and fragmentation of the bone.

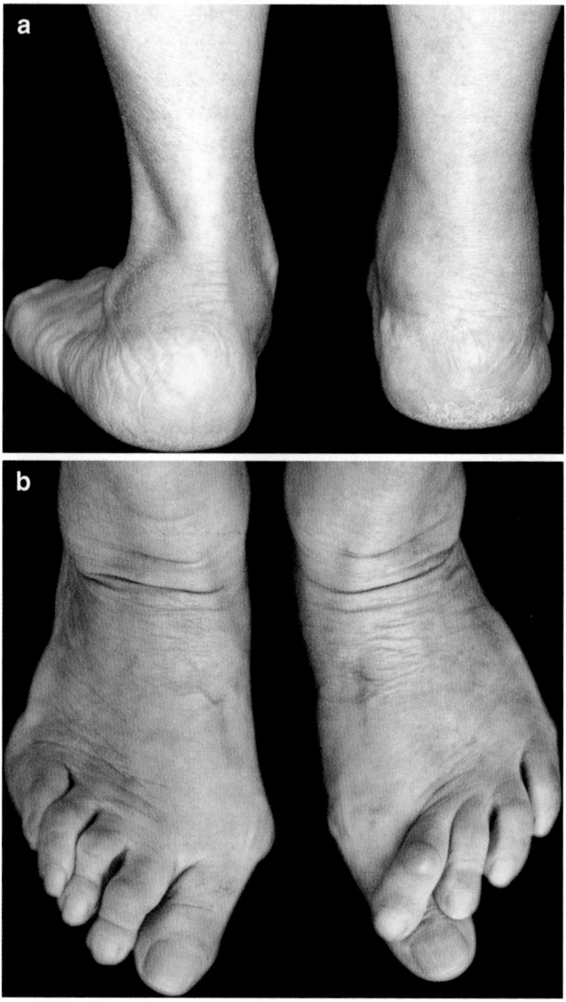

FIGURE 4.23 Common foot deformities in patients with rheumatoid arthritis. (**a**) Calcaneus valgus. (**b**) Triangular forefoot (hallux valgus and medial deviation of the other toes)

Treatment should be prophylactic, based on careful control of the diabetes, comfortable shoes and regular visits to the doctor and footcare specialist or chiropodist.

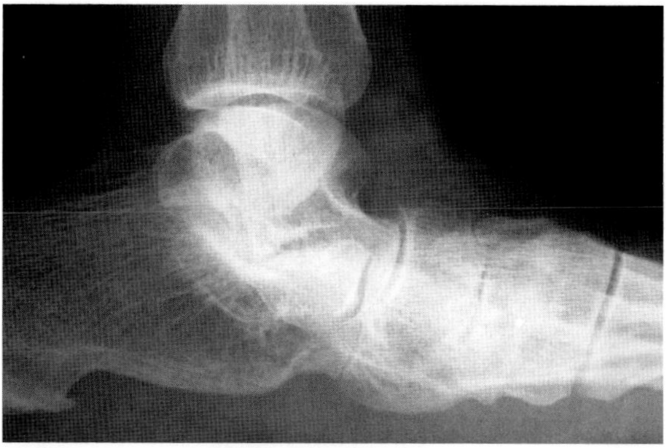

FIGURE 4.24 Rheumatoid foot. Collapse of the talonavicular joint resulting in secondary flat foot

Complex Regional Pain Syndrome (Reflex Sympathetic Dystrophy, Algodystrophy, etc.)

The foot is the most common location of this relatively rare, but interesting and potentially incapacitating condition. It results from a regional deregulation of the sympathetic nervous system that leads to persistent, chronic vasodilation. Left untreated, this conditions leads to atrophy of the bones, muscles and skin and retraction of the soft tissue.

It may affect several joints, especially the feet, knees, hands and hips (where it is sometimes called "transient osteoporosis of the hip").

It often appears after major or minor trauma. In the hands, it is a common complication of Colles' fractures or surgical procedures but may also follow myocardial infarction (Dressler's shoulder-hand syndrome).

The patient usually describes diffuse severe pain, usually unilateral, with a variable rhythm, which can go from being typically inflammatory to characteristically mechanical. The onset is insidious, with progressive deterioration that may reach total functional disability of the affected area.

In the initial stages, the affected area normally presents diffuse swelling with pitting, which extends beyond the limits of

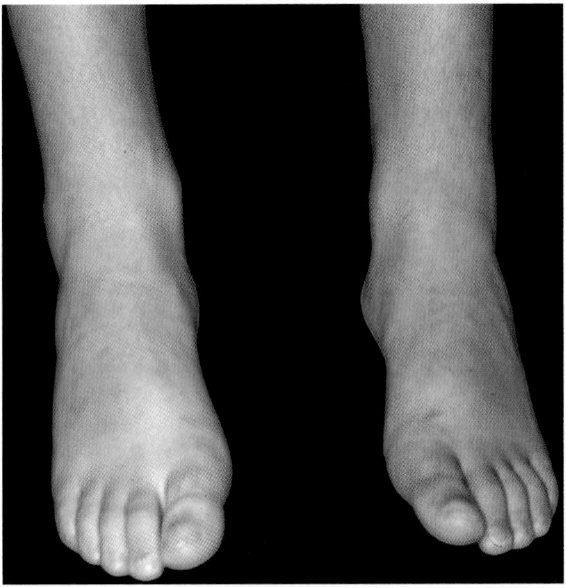

FIGURE 4.25 Algodystrophy in a 12 year old boy. Diffuse swelling of the foot which gains a purple discoloration when dependent. (Courtesy: Dr. Manuel Salgado.)

the joints. There is diffuse purplish coloring, exacerbated by a long period with the limbs dependent. There may be clear difference in temperature (warmer in the initial phases, colder in later stages) and perspiration may be more accentuated on the affected side (Fig. 4.25). Absence of these vasomotor signs makes diagnosis more difficult, particularly in deep joints.

With time, these suggestive vasomotor changes can become discreet. The diagnosis then depends on a strong clinical suspicion, the enquiry and a thorough physical examination.

Plain films may be normal, but sometimes present a typical patchy osteopenia – Fig. 4.26. Tecnethium bone scanning can also be helpful. For a long time, increased uptake of the radioligand will predominate with a diffuse appearance, extending beyond the limits of the joint (Fig. 4.27). Diffuse increased uptake in the foot is common and involves several joints of the tarsus. Early scintigraphic images, in the first few

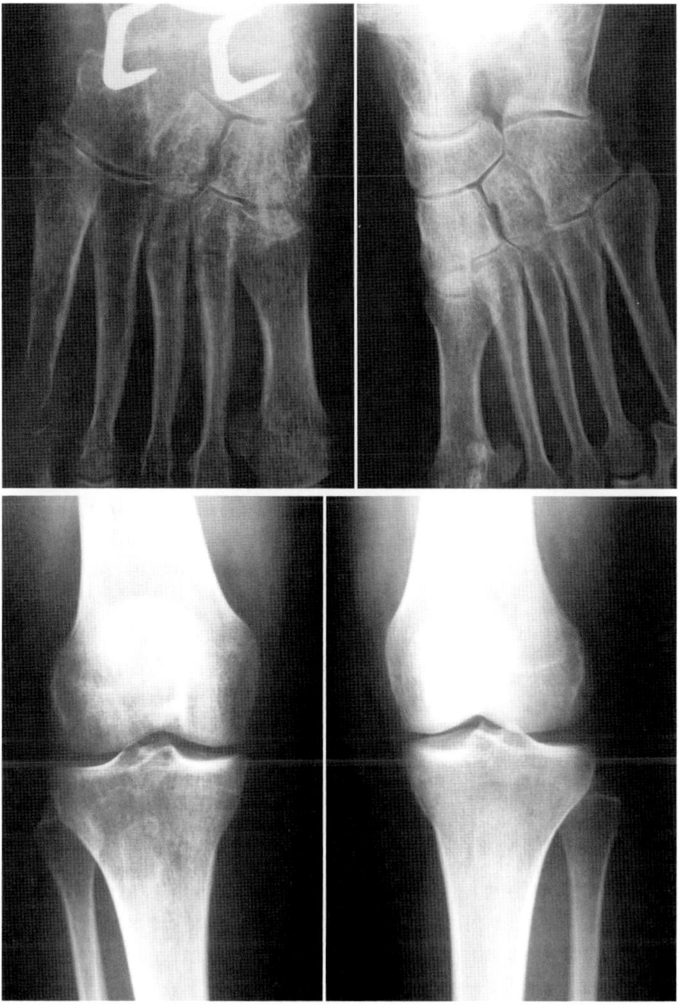

FIGURE 4.26 Algodystrophy. The right foot was affected following a surgical procedure. The patient suffering from the right knee described a minor trauma 4 months before (vd. bone scintigraphy of this patient – Fig. 4.27)

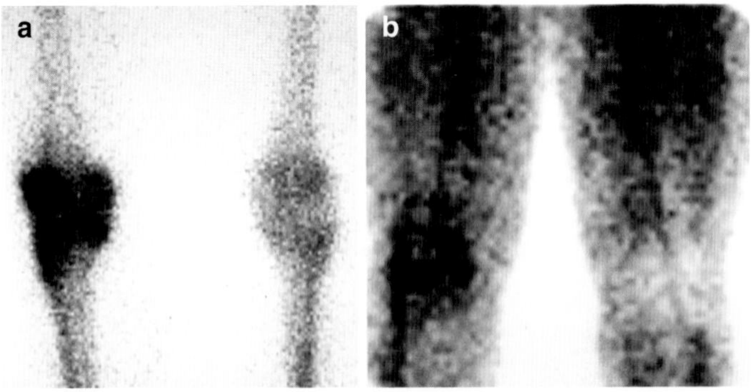

FIGURE 4.27 Algodystrophy of the right knee. Late phase cintigraphy images (bone phase - 2–3 hours after injection of the tracer) show increased uptake of the radiotracer. The diffuse distribution and the extension of bone activity beyond the joint suggest algodystrophy but are not specific (**a**). Hyperfixation in the early phase (vascular phase - first few minutes after injection) is a stronger suggestion of this condition but still not specific (**b**)

minutes (the vascular phase), can reinforce the diagnosis if they show an increase in local radioactivity. Conversely, in the later stages, there may be regional decreased uptake of the radioligand. The patient's sedimentation rate remains normal.

Treatment becomes less effective over time. If not properly treated, the condition may develop into marked atrophy and retraction of the subcutaneous and muscular tissue, with total, irreversible functional disability (Sudeck's atrophy).

If the clinical picture supports a reasonable suspicion of this condition, the patient should be urgently referred to a specialist.

Treatment

In general practice the vast majority of cases of pain limited to the foot will have mechanical cause. Treatment basically consists of correcting functional anomalies and relieving the load on the feet, by changing the patient's footwear and weight.

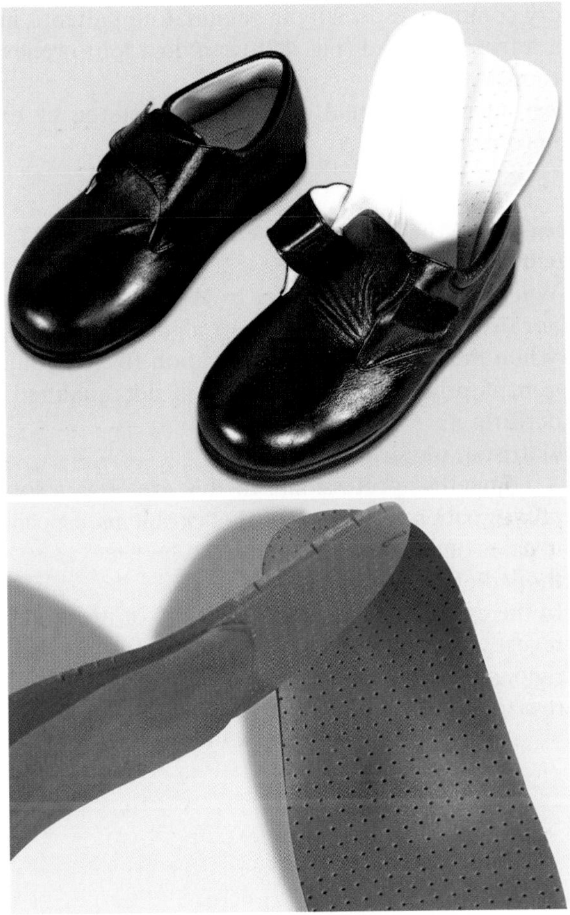

FIGURE 4.28 Patients with foot deformities should be advised to wear well-fitted, capacious, cushioned shoes with thick flexible rubbery soles Insoles with a thickened bar just behind the metatarsophalangeal joints help relieve pressure and pain in this area

The services of qualified specialists in orthosis and podiatry are invaluable in more difficult cases. A careful choice of footwear or even custom-made shoes can be extremely useful in relieving these patients' pain (Fig. 4.28). If there are painful calluses under the heads of the metatarsals, which are very common, especially in rheumatoid patients, insoles with a retrocapital pad (Fig. 4.28) can do a lot to relieve the symptoms.

Local injections should only be administered by experienced professionals.

When Should The Patient Be Referred To A Specialist?

Rheumatologist:

- Whenever there are reasons to suspect arthritis, seronegative spondylarthropathy or algodystrophy;
- When there is a probable indication for local injection, if primary care physician is not qualified to perform it.

Podiatrist or physical therapist:

- A competent professional in this area has a lot to offer a patient with serious foot problems, especially in cases of deformity or calluses.

Orthopedic surgeon:

- In the case of accentuated instability of the ankle or severe deformity of the feet (hallux valgus, hallux rigidus, flat or arched feet), with functional disability resistant to conservative measures.

Index

J.A.P. da Silva, A.D. Woolf, *Rheumatology of the Lower Limbs in Clinical Practice*, DOI 10.1007/978-1-4471-2253-1,